Personal Medical Journal

If I have misplaced this journal, please contact me or forward it to the following:

Name _____

I0486272

Address _____

_____

Phone ( ) _____

E-mail _____

Date: _____ From _____ To _____

Emergency Numbers

1. _____ _____ _____

2. _____ _____ _____

3. _____ _____ _____

4. _____ _____ _____

5. _____ _____ _____

Acknowledgements

A special thank you.

To my children — Laurie, Michael and Jill, who gave me the inspiration to use a similar book throughout their childhood. It continues to be an important tool for their continuum of health care and assists many medical professionals especially when emergencies have arisen, even into their adulthood.

To my late husband, Norman Cordle, who offered encouragement. My family—Richard and Sally Lopez, and my Mother, Amparo Lopez, who have always been a tremendous source of support and strength. To Judith and Michele Troutman who have stood by me and assisted with recommendations.

Also, to the many families, medical and educational professionals, and friends who have asked for this book and who have provided the encouragement and enthusiasm that helped make it a reality.

~ Gloria Ann Lopez

PERSONAL MEDICAL JOURNAL

GLORIA ANN LOPEZ

The Journey of One's Heart

The journey of one's heart

is a path to richness and fulfillment.

The truth for which we seek is always there in front of us.

The beauty we experience is the beauty from within.

The light is constant upon our everlasting self.

The love we receive is a mere reflection of what we offer.

The path we experience is our journey of truth and self-growth.

The strength we show comes from the One Source.

Be gentle with your spirit.

Gloria Ann Lopez

CONTENTS

How To Manage Your Medical History

This *Personal Medical Journal* has been proven to be a lifesaver. It will assist you by managing your own health history, that of a child or of another individual throughout his or her life. You will find this very useful when you go to the doctor's office or if you have a serious medical situation. Take this journal with you, especially while you are traveling and away from home, in case you require medical treatment. It will provide an overview of your medical history to assist the medical professional.

Sectioned into various categories, the Personal Medical Journal is a notebook to assist you when you visit a physician, dentist, therapist, hospital, or any service agency. You can tailor it for your individual needs, or that of an individual you are caring for by taking your own notes and adding your own style. This is YOUR journal and the format presented is to assist you.

To aid you further with your health management, ask your physician, dentist, and any medical professional you visit for a copy of their report for your files. This can include the following: copies of any x-ray, laboratory studies, special procedures, surgical, and special testing reports. Add any information that you feel is important to you and/or will be helpful to another physician, therapist or a service provider.

For your convenience, there is an emergency card in the back of this book for you to fill out and keep in your wallet.

Purchase a 3-ring binder and dividers from your local supermarket, office supply store, or pharmacy. Dividers sectioned into the different disciplines/ fields of service you are working with (i.e. Neurosurgery, Surgical Reports, X-ray Reports, Psychological Reports, Physician Summaries, Laboratory Results/Reports, etc.) will make it easier to locate information. If you are maintaining a file for a child, include copies of the Individual Educational Programs (IEP) and similar school reports.

Request copies of your x-ray films for your permanent files. They can be used as a comparison and/or provide necessary information needed for a treatment. These can prove to be invaluable. If you have several physicians you visit, or when you are traveling, be sure to take the pertinent information with you. The x-ray films fit perfectly in an art portfolio that is available at your local art supply store.

If you have special needs or you are a caregiver for such an individual make a video on what is needed for care. Include feeding, bathing, cooking, transfer techniques, and personal care. As well as where items need to be located in the kitchen, bathroom, and the house, and notes to assist other caregivers and/or attendants. If the x-ray films are available, you can tape them to a window with some type of light behind them, so while you are videotaping you will be able to explain the medical situation. Also, if there is equipment required this is the perfect opportunity to explain how to use it, what areas of concern require special attention, type of maintenance, and any other information. This provides a continuum of care to enhance the quality of life of an individual and helps eliminate the repetition of information. Look for my upcoming book for caregivers to assist a person with long-term care needs and to maintain stabilized medical care.

The following page is a general overview of each section within the Personal Medical Journal.

Consider your journal as a tool to assist you and as you use it you will no longer need to memorize every detail regarding your medical history. The professional is generally pleased to see you are organized and have the information they need for your optimum care.

Congratulations! You now have the comfort of self-reliance and accuracy with your medical history.

MANAGEMENT INSTRUCTIONS

Enjoy the peace of mind!

❧

GLORIA ANN LOPEZ

Medical History: An overview to assist with the general questions asked. State any diagnosis or any corrective procedure that has occurred during your lifetime.

Mother's Pregnancy History: Especially important for children as these questions will come up for years.

Allergies: Medication and Foods — *Critical Section — Write down any reactions, and what medication or treatment was necessary to resolve the allergic reaction, etc. This is extremely important for any medical professional who is assisting you.

Medication Log: It is important to keep a record of all your prescriptions, over-the-counter and herbal medications to better assist medical professionals.

Medication Records: Information on the medications you are taking.

Medication Daily Schedule: If there are several pill-form medications taken daily, it is suggested to ask the pharmacist if they will prepare a bubble pack for the medications. If this is not available through your local pharmacy, then purchase a weekly Sunday through Saturday plastic holder (some pharmacies will give these away at no additional cost, so ask your pharmacist). It is recommended that you purchase a minimum of 3 to 4 boxes of different sizes and/or colors, in order to easily distinquish the time the medication is scheduled to be taken.

Place the medication in the appropriate box organized by time of day. If possible, check with the physician and/or pharmacist regarding information on which pills can or cannot be taken at the same time.

- i.e. Morning, Noon, Dinner, Evening/Bedtime, Other (if applicable) such as aspirin type, sleeping pills, etc.

Alerts — Concerns: Write any health and/or medical concerns that occur, or areas that need to be continually observed.

Hospitalizations * **Surgeries** * **Procedures:** You, the physician, or the dentist can summarize the procedure, complications, and any notes in this area. Ask for a copy of his/her notes for your file/binder.

Medical Appointments * **Doctor Visits:** Write the reason for the visit (routine, emergency, etc). This is especially helpful to keep abreast of what has occurred, and for a continuum of health. You can have the doctor summarize the procedure, complications, and any notes in this area. If you feel it is needed, ask the doctor for a copy of his/her notes for your file/binder.

Dental Appointments: This is especially helpful for your dentist when you are referred to a specialist or another dentist.

Laboratory Work * **X-ray:** State the type of test, the reason for it and the results. Depending on the test, request a copy of the report and/or x-ray for your file. This is helpful especially for future reference and to assist any professional when evaluating a medical treatment or condition. If the service provider will not release the report to you, you will need to request that it be sent to your physician. Then you can request a copy from your physician.

Immunizations: These records will be needed throughout your lifetime.

Academic Programs * **Service Agencies:** If you are utilizing the services of a special program, association or provider, it will be helpful to have the information available to share with your professional team.

Names and Addresses Index: Keep the phone numbers and addresses of any one who is assisting you with your medical / dental health care.

MANAGEMENT INSTRUCTIONS

Note: If you do not need a section at this time, remove it and save it for future use. Remember, this is your Personal Medical Journal, feel free to customize it for your needs.

A Day Of Sunshine

A day of sunshine is merely a breath of fresh air

The beauty surrounding

The vision to capsulate

The evening of solitude

The stars to complete the wonder

of life and the beauty within.

Gloria Ann Lopez

Medical History
Mother's Pregnancy History

Medical History: An overview to assist with the general questions asked. State any diagnosis or any corrective procedure that has occurred during your lifetime.

Mother's Pregnancy History: Especially important for children as these questions will come up for years.

Personal Information

Name _____

Address _____

City _____ State_____

Country _____ Zip _____

Phone (   ) _____ Fax (   ) _____

Work (   ) _____ Cell (   ) _____

Email _____ Religion _____

S.S.# xxx-xx-_____ DOB _____ Blood Type _____

Ethnic Background_____

Children # _____ Ages_____

Nearest Relative Name_____

Relationship_____ Phone (   ) _____

Other Phone (   ) _____

Family History

❏   (Attach separate sheet with more information.)

	Date	Diagnosis	Relative	Comment
1.				
2.				
3.				
4.				
5.				
6.				

Comments: _____

_____

_____

_____

Physicians / Dentists

(Place full address information in address section. It is recommended that you obtain the business card and place it in the plastic holder for easy reference.)

Date	Doctor	Phone	Specialty
1.			
2.			
3.			
4.			
5.			
6.			

Insurance Information

(It is recommended that you place a copy of your insurance cards in the plastic business card holder for easy reference.)

Medicare # _____ Medical # _____

Other Type _____ No. _____

Subscriber _____

Subscriber No. _____ Effective _____

Medical Insurance: Carrier_____

Group No._____

Member Services Phone No.(   ) _____

Co-Pay $_____Office $ _____ Hosp. $ _____

Emerg. $_____Rx $ _____ Other $ _____

Primary Physician _____

Plan Code_____

Employer _____

Address_____Phone (   )_____

Dental: Carrier _____ Plan # _____

Member Services Phone No. (   ) _____ Co-Pay_____

Other Coverage _____

NOTE_____

© 2008 Life Cycles Publishing, Inc. All Rights Reserved.

Additional Information

Specific notations:

- **Allergies:** ☐ Latex ☐ Penicillin ☐ Iodine ☐ Metal ☐ Others: see list
- **Phobias:** ☐ Shots / Needles ☐ Dental ☐ Other _____
- **Reflex notation:** ☐ Gag ☐ Other _____
- **Prothesis / Implants: Type**
  - ☐ Dentures ☐ Fixed ☐ Removable ☐ Full ☐ Partial
  - ☐ Body ☐ External _____
  - ☐ Internal _____
- **Heart Pacemaker**

(Please use for additional information.)

_____

_____

_____

_____

_____

_____

_____

_____

_____

_____

_____

_____

_____

_____

_____

_____

_____

Mother's Pregnancy History

This is especially important for children as these questions will come up for years.

MOTHER'S PREGNANCY HISTORY

Mother's Pregnancy History

(Please use the next page for notes or any questions/concerns.)

Child's Name _____

Mother's Name _____ Father's Name _____

Pregnancy Term ❑ Full ❑ Other _____

❑ Fertility: *Attach separate note* ❑ Rh Factor: *(See Medication section)*

Tests

Date	Type	Results	Complications

Medications

Date	Type	Dosage	Frequency	Purpose

DELIVERY: Date_____Time_____ Labor Time _____

❑ Cesarean Section ❑ Natural ❑ Epidural ❑ Other _____

❑ Complications ❑ Mother ❑ Baby Explain_____

_____

❑ Baby: ❑ Multiple # _____ Explain _____

_____

Mother's Pregnancy History Notes

Additional Information

(Please use for additional information.)

_____

_____

_____

_____

_____

_____

_____

_____

_____

_____

_____

_____

_____

_____

_____

_____

_____

_____

_____

_____

_____

_____

_____

_____

Allergy List
Allergy Record

Allergies: Medication and Foods — *Critical Section Write down any reactions, and what medication or treatment was necessary to resolve the allergic reaction, etc. This is extremely important for any medical professional who is assisting you.

Notes

Allergies

Allergy List

❏ MEDICATION   ❏ FOOD   ❏ OTHER
(Best to use a separate page for each category.)

	Name	Date	Reaction
1.			
2.			
3.			
4.			
5.			
6.			
7.			
8.			
9.			
10.			
11.			
12.			
13.			
14.			
15.			

Allergies

Allergy List

❏ **MEDICATION**   ❏ **FOOD**   ❏ **OTHER**
(Best to use a separate page for each category.)

	Name	Date	Reaction
1.			
2.			
3.			
4.			
5.			
6.			
7.			
8.			
9.			
10.			
11.			
12.			
13.			
14.			
15.			

Allergies

Allergy List

❏ **MEDICATION**　　❏ **FOOD**　　❏ **OTHER**
(Best to use a separate page for each category.)

	Name	Date	Reaction
1.			
2.			
3.			
4.			
5.			
6.			
7.			
8.			
9.			
10.			
11.			
12.			
13.			
14.			
15.			

Allergies

Allergy List

❏ **MEDICATION**   ❏ **FOOD**   ❏ **OTHER**
(Best to use a separate page for each category.)

Allergies

	Name	Date	Reaction
1.			
2.			
3.			
4.			
5.			
6.			
7.			
8.			
9.			
10.			
11.			
12.			
13.			
14.			
15.			

Allergy List

❏ MEDICATION   ❏ FOOD   ❏ OTHER
(Best to use a separate page for each category.)

	Name	Date	Reaction
1.			
2.			
3.			
4.			
5.			
6.			
7.			
8.			
9.			
10.			
11.			
12.			
13.			
14.			
15.			

Allergies

Allergy List

❏ **MEDICATION**   ❏ **FOOD**   ❏ **OTHER**
(Best to use a separate page for each category.)

	Name	Date	Reaction
1.			
2.			
3.			
4.			
5.			
6.			
7.			
8.			
9.			
10.			
11.			
12.			
13.			
14.			
15.			

Allergy Records

(Best to use a separate page for each category.)

Date _____

Name _____

Dosage _____

Reaction _____

_____

_____

Physician _____

Counteraction _____

_____

Date _____

Name _____

Dosage _____

Reaction _____

_____

_____

Physician _____

Counteraction _____

_____

Date _____

Name _____

Dosage _____

Reaction _____

_____

_____

Physician _____

Counteraction _____

_____

Allergies

Allergy Records

❑ **MEDICATION** ❑ **FOOD** ❑ **OTHER**

(Best to use a separate page for each category.)

Date ______________________________

Name ______________________________

Dosage ______________________________

Reaction ______________________________

____

____

Physician ______________________________

Counteraction ______________________________

____

Date ______________________________

Name ______________________________

Dosage ______________________________

Reaction ______________________________

____

____

Physician ______________________________

Counteraction ______________________________

____

Date ______________________________

Name ______________________________

Dosage ______________________________

Reaction ______________________________

____

____

Physician ______________________________

Counteraction ______________________________

____

Allergies

Allergy Records

❏ MEDICATION   ❏ FOOD   ❏ OTHER
(Best to use a separate page for each category.)

Date _____

Name _____

Dosage _____

Reaction _____

_____

_____

Physician _____

Counteraction _____

_____

Date _____

Name _____

Dosage _____

Reaction _____

_____

_____

Physician _____

Counteraction _____

_____

Date _____

Name _____

Dosage _____

Reaction _____

_____

_____

Physician _____

Counteraction _____

_____

Allergies

Allergy Records

❏ **MEDICATION**   ❏ **FOOD**   ❏ **OTHER**
(Best to use a separate page for each category.)

Date _____

Name _____

Dosage _____

Reaction _____

_____

_____

Physician _____

Counteraction _____

_____

Date _____

Name _____

Dosage _____

Reaction _____

_____

_____

Physician _____

Counteraction _____

_____

Date _____

Name _____

Dosage _____

Reaction _____

_____

_____

Physician _____

Counteraction _____

_____

Allergies

Allergy Records

❏ **MEDICATION**   ❏ **FOOD**   ❏ **OTHER**
(Best to use a separate page for each category.)

Date _____

Name _____

Dosage _____

Reaction _____

_____

_____

Physician _____

Counteraction _____

_____

Date _____

Name _____

Dosage _____

Reaction _____

_____

_____

Physician _____

Counteraction _____

_____

Date _____

Name _____

Dosage _____

Reaction _____

_____

_____

Physician _____

Counteraction _____

_____

Allergies

Allergy Records

❏ **MEDICATION**   ❏ **FOOD**   ❏ **OTHER**
(Best to use a separate page for each category.)

Date _____

Name _____

Dosage _____

Reaction _____

_____

_____

Physician _____

Counteraction _____

_____

Date _____

Name _____

Dosage _____

Reaction _____

_____

_____

Physician _____

Counteraction _____

_____

Date _____

Name _____

Dosage _____

Reaction _____

_____

_____

Physician _____

Counteraction _____

_____

Allergies

Medication Log
Medication Records
Medication Daily Schedule

Medication Log: It is important to keep a record of all your prescriptions, over-the-counter and herbal medications to better assist medical professionals.

Medication Records: Information on the medications you are taking.

Medication Daily Schedule: If there are several pill-form medications taken daily, it is suggested to ask the pharmacist if they will prepare a bubble pack for the medications. If this is not available through your local pharmacy, then purchase a weekly Sunday through Saturday plastic holder (some pharmacies will give these away at no additional cost, so ask your pharmacist). It is recommended that you purchase a minimum of 3 to 4 boxes of different sizes and/or colors, in order to easily distinquish the time the medication is scheduled to be taken.

Place the medication in the appropriate box organized by time of day. If possible, check with the physician and/or pharmacist regarding information on which pills can or cannot be taken at the same time.

- i.e. Morning, Noon, Dinner, Evening/Bedtime, Other (if applicable) such as aspirin type, sleeping pills, etc.

Medications

Notes

Medications

Medication Log

Maintain a log/list on your medications for easy access.

Place a:

(✓) or **date** in Reaction when symptoms occur then explain in "Allergy: Medication."

(✓) or **date** at the *Stopped* Section when finished taking your medication.

DATE	DRUG or APPLICATION	DOSAGE	FREQUENCY	REACTION *See Allergy Section	OTHER	STOPPED/DISCONTINUED	COMMENTS

Medications

Medication Log

Maintain a log/list on your medications for easy access.

Place a:

(✓) or **date** in Reaction when symptoms occur then explain in "Allergy: Medication."

(✓) or **date** at the *Stopped* Section when finished taking your medication.

DATE	DRUG or APPLICATION	DOSAGE	FREQUENCY	REACTION *See Allergy Section	OTHER	STOPPED/DISCONTINUED	COMMENTS

Medications

Medication Log

Maintain a log/list on your medications for easy access.

Place a:

(✓) or **date** in Reaction when symptoms occur then explain in "Allergy: Medication."

(✓) or **date** at the *Stopped* Section when finished taking your medication.

DATE	DRUG or APPLICATION	DOSAGE	FREQUENCY	REACTION *See Allergy Section	OTHER	STOPPED/DISCONTINUED	COMMENTS

Medications

Medication Log

Maintain a log/list on your medications for easy access.

Place a:

(✓) or **date** in Reaction when symptoms occur then explain in "Allergy: Medication."

(✓) or **date** at the *Stopped* Section when finished taking your medication.

DATE	DRUG or APPLICATION	DOSAGE	FREQUENCY	REACTION *See Allergy Section	OTHER	STOPPED/DISCONTINUED	COMMENTS

Medications

Medication Log

Maintain a log/list on your medications for easy access.

Place a:

(✓) or **date** in Reaction when symptoms occur then explain in "Allergy: Medication."

(✓) or **date** at the *Stopped* Section when finished taking your medication.

DATE	DRUG or APPLICATION	DOSAGE	FREQUENCY	REACTION *See Allergy Section	OTHER	STOPPED/DISCONTINUED	COMMENTS

Medications

Medication Log

Maintain a log/list on your medications for easy access.

Place a:

(✓) or **date** in Reaction when symptoms occur then explain in "Allergy: Medication."

(✓) or **date** at the *Stopped* Section when finished taking your medication.

DATE	DRUG or APPLICATION	DOSAGE	FREQUENCY	REACTION *See Allergy Section	OTHER	STOPPED/DISCONTINUED	COMMENTS

Medications

Medication Records

Date _____ Dr. _____ Phone _____

Medication _____ Rx.# _____

Purpose _____

Dosage: _____mg _____ length *(days)* Other _____

Time:
				Other

Special Instructions *(i.e., taken with food, increase water, etc.)* _____

_____

Side effects (i.e., may cause drowsiness, etc.)_____

_____

Discontinued: Date _____   ❏ Monthly prescription refill

Reason ❏ Completed   ❏ Reaction: *Be sure to add to Allergy-Medication Section.*

Date _____ Dr. _____ Phone _____

Medication _____ Rx.# _____

Purpose _____

Dosage: _____mg _____ length *(days)* Other _____

Time:
				Other

Special Instructions *(i.e., taken with food, increase water, etc.)* _____

_____

Side effects (i.e., may cause drowsiness, etc.)_____

_____

Discontinued: Date _____   ❏ Monthly prescription refill

Reason ❏ Completed   ❏ Reaction: *Be sure to add to Allergy-Medication Section.*

Date _____ Dr. _____ Phone _____

Medication _____ Rx.# _____

Purpose _____

Dosage: _____mg _____ length *(days)* Other _____

Time:
				Other

Special Instructions *(i.e., taken with food, increase water, etc.)* _____

_____

Side effects (i.e., may cause drowsiness, etc.)_____

_____

Discontinued: Date _____   ❏ Monthly prescription refill

Reason ❏ Completed   ❏ Reaction: *Be sure to add to Allergy-Medication Section.*

Medications

Medication Records

Date _____ Dr. _____ Phone _____
Medication _____ Rx.# _____
Purpose _____
Dosage: _____mg _____ length *(days)*   Other _____

Time:					Other

Special Instructions *(i.e., taken with food, increase water, etc.)* _____
_____

Side effects (i.e., may cause drowsiness, etc.)_____
_____

Discontinued: Date _____   ❏ Monthly prescription refill
Reason ❏ Completed   ❏ Reaction: *Be sure to add to Allergy-Medication Section.*

Date _____ Dr. _____ Phone _____
Medication _____ Rx.# _____
Purpose _____
Dosage: _____mg _____ length *(days)*   Other _____

Time:					Other

Special Instructions *(i.e., taken with food, increase water, etc.)* _____
_____

Side effects (i.e., may cause drowsiness, etc.)_____
_____

Discontinued: Date _____   ❏ Monthly prescription refill
Reason ❏ Completed   ❏ Reaction: *Be sure to add to Allergy-Medication Section.*

Date _____ Dr. _____ Phone _____
Medication _____ Rx.# _____
Purpose _____
Dosage: _____mg _____ length *(days)*   Other _____

Time:					Other

Special Instructions *(i.e., taken with food, increase water, etc.)* _____
_____

Side effects (i.e., may cause drowsiness, etc.)_____
_____

Discontinued: Date _____   ❏ Monthly prescription refill
Reason ❏ Completed   ❏ Reaction: *Be sure to add to Allergy-Medication Section.*

Medications

Medication Records

Date _____ Dr. _____ Phone _____

Medication _____ Rx.# _____

Purpose _____

Dosage: _____mg _____ length *(days)* Other _____

Time:

				Other

Special Instructions *(i.e., taken with food, increase water, etc.)* _____

_____

Side effects (i.e., may cause drowsiness, etc.)_____

_____

Discontinued: Date _____   ❑ Monthly prescription refill

Reason ❑ Completed   ❑ Reaction: *Be sure to add to Allergy-Medication Section.*

Date _____ Dr. _____ Phone _____

Medication _____ Rx.# _____

Purpose _____

Dosage: _____mg _____ length *(days)* Other _____

Time:

				Other

Special Instructions *(i.e., taken with food, increase water, etc.)* _____

_____

Side effects (i.e., may cause drowsiness, etc.)_____

_____

Discontinued: Date _____   ❑ Monthly prescription refill

Reason ❑ Completed   ❑ Reaction: *Be sure to add to Allergy-Medication Section.*

Date _____ Dr. _____ Phone _____

Medication _____ Rx.# _____

Purpose _____

Dosage: _____mg _____ length *(days)* Other _____

Time:

				Other

Special Instructions *(i.e., taken with food, increase water, etc.)* _____

_____

Side effects (i.e., may cause drowsiness, etc.)_____

_____

Discontinued: Date _____   ❑ Monthly prescription refill

Reason ❑ Completed   ❑ Reaction: *Be sure to add to Allergy-Medication Section.*

Medications

Medication Records

Date _____ Dr. _____ Phone _____

Medication _____ Rx.# _____

Purpose _____

Dosage: _____mg _____ length *(days)*   Other _____

Time:					Other

Special Instructions *(i.e., taken with food, increase water, etc.)* _____

_____

Side effects (i.e., may cause drowsiness, etc.)_____

_____

Discontinued: Date _____   ❏ Monthly prescription refill

Reason ❏ Completed   ❏ Reaction: *Be sure to add to Allergy-Medication Section.*

Date _____ Dr. _____ Phone _____

Medication _____ Rx.# _____

Purpose _____

Dosage: _____mg _____ length *(days)*   Other _____

Time:					Other

Special Instructions *(i.e., taken with food, increase water, etc.)* _____

_____

Side effects (i.e., may cause drowsiness, etc.)_____

_____

Discontinued: Date _____   ❏ Monthly prescription refill

Reason ❏ Completed   ❏ Reaction: *Be sure to add to Allergy-Medication Section.*

Date _____ Dr. _____ Phone _____

Medication _____ Rx.# _____

Purpose _____

Dosage: _____mg _____ length *(days)*   Other _____

Time:					Other

Special Instructions *(i.e., taken with food, increase water, etc.)* _____

_____

Side effects (i.e., may cause drowsiness, etc.)_____

_____

Discontinued: Date _____   ❏ Monthly prescription refill

Reason ❏ Completed   ❏ Reaction: *Be sure to add to Allergy-Medication Section.*

Medications

Medication Records

Date _____ Dr. _____ Phone _____

Medication _____ Rx.# _____

Purpose _____

Dosage: _____ mg _____ length *(days)*   Other _____

Time:

				Other

Special Instructions *(i.e., taken with food, increase water, etc.)* _____

_____

Side effects (i.e., may cause drowsiness, etc.)_____

_____

Discontinued: Date _____   ❏ Monthly prescription refill

Reason ❏ Completed   ❏ Reaction: *Be sure to add to Allergy-Medication Section.*

Date _____ Dr. _____ Phone _____

Medication _____ Rx.# _____

Purpose _____

Dosage: _____ mg _____ length *(days)*   Other _____

Time:

				Other

Special Instructions *(i.e., taken with food, increase water, etc.)* _____

_____

Side effects (i.e., may cause drowsiness, etc.)_____

_____

Discontinued: Date _____   ❏ Monthly prescription refill

Reason ❏ Completed   ❏ Reaction: *Be sure to add to Allergy-Medication Section.*

Date _____ Dr. _____ Phone _____

Medication _____ Rx.# _____

Purpose _____

Dosage: _____ mg _____ length *(days)*   Other _____

Time:

				Other

Special Instructions *(i.e., taken with food, increase water, etc.)* _____

_____

Side effects (i.e., may cause drowsiness, etc.)_____

_____

Discontinued: Date _____   ❏ Monthly prescription refill

Reason ❏ Completed   ❏ Reaction: *Be sure to add to Allergy-Medication Section.*

Medications

Medication Records

Date _____ Dr. _____ Phone _____

Medication _____ Rx.# _____

Purpose _____

Dosage: _____mg _____ length *(days)*   Other _____

Time:					Other

Special Instructions *(i.e., taken with food, increase water, etc.)* _____

_____

Side effects (i.e., may cause drowsiness, etc.)_____

_____

Discontinued: Date _____   ❏ Monthly prescription refill

Reason ❏ Completed   ❏ Reaction: *Be sure to add to Allergy-Medication Section.*

Date _____ Dr. _____ Phone _____

Medication _____ Rx.# _____

Purpose _____

Dosage: _____mg _____ length *(days)*   Other _____

Time:					Other

Special Instructions *(i.e., taken with food, increase water, etc.)* _____

_____

Side effects (i.e., may cause drowsiness, etc.)_____

_____

Discontinued: Date _____   ❏ Monthly prescription refill

Reason ❏ Completed   ❏ Reaction: *Be sure to add to Allergy-Medication Section.*

Date _____ Dr. _____ Phone _____

Medication _____ Rx.# _____

Purpose _____

Dosage: _____mg _____ length *(days)*   Other _____

Time:					Other

Special Instructions *(i.e., taken with food, increase water, etc.)* _____

_____

Side effects (i.e., may cause drowsiness, etc.)_____

_____

Discontinued: Date _____   ❏ Monthly prescription refill

Reason ❏ Completed   ❏ Reaction: *Be sure to add to Allergy-Medication Section.*

Medications

Medication Records

Date _____ Dr. _____ Phone _____

Medication _____ Rx.# _____

Purpose _____

Dosage: _____mg _____ length *(days)*   Other _____

Time:

				Other

Special Instructions *(i.e., taken with food, increase water, etc.)* _____

_____

Side effects (i.e., may cause drowsiness, etc.)_____

_____

Discontinued: Date _____   ❑ Monthly prescription refill

Reason ❑ Completed   ❑ Reaction: *Be sure to add to Allergy-Medication Section.*

Date _____ Dr. _____ Phone _____

Medication _____ Rx.# _____

Purpose _____

Dosage: _____mg _____ length *(days)*   Other _____

Time:

				Other

Special Instructions *(i.e., taken with food, increase water, etc.)* _____

_____

Side effects (i.e., may cause drowsiness, etc.)_____

_____

Discontinued: Date _____   ❑ Monthly prescription refill

Reason ❑ Completed   ❑ Reaction: *Be sure to add to Allergy-Medication Section.*

Date _____ Dr. _____ Phone _____

Medication _____ Rx.# _____

Purpose _____

Dosage: _____mg _____ length *(days)*   Other _____

Time:

				Other

Special Instructions *(i.e., taken with food, increase water, etc.)* _____

_____

Side effects (i.e., may cause drowsiness, etc.)_____

_____

Discontinued: Date _____   ❑ Monthly prescription refill

Reason ❑ Completed   ❑ Reaction: *Be sure to add to Allergy-Medication Section.*

Medications

Medication Records

Date _____ Dr. _____ Phone _____

Medication _____ Rx.# _____

Purpose _____

Dosage: _____mg _____ length *(days)*   Other _____

Time:					Other

Special Instructions *(i.e., taken with food, increase water, etc.)* _____

_____

Side effects (i.e., may cause drowsiness, etc.)_____

_____

Discontinued: Date _____   ❏ Monthly prescription refill

Reason ❏ Completed   ❏ Reaction: *Be sure to add to Allergy-Medication Section.*

Date _____ Dr. _____ Phone _____

Medication _____ Rx.# _____

Purpose _____

Dosage: _____mg _____ length *(days)*   Other _____

Time:					Other

Special Instructions *(i.e., taken with food, increase water, etc.)* _____

_____

Side effects (i.e., may cause drowsiness, etc.)_____

_____

Discontinued: Date _____   ❏ Monthly prescription refill

Reason ❏ Completed   ❏ Reaction: *Be sure to add to Allergy-Medication Section.*

Date _____ Dr. _____ Phone _____

Medication _____ Rx.# _____

Purpose _____

Dosage: _____mg _____ length *(days)*   Other _____

Time:					Other

Special Instructions *(i.e., taken with food, increase water, etc.)* _____

_____

Side effects (i.e., may cause drowsiness, etc.)_____

_____

Discontinued: Date _____   ❏ Monthly prescription refill

Reason ❏ Completed   ❏ Reaction: *Be sure to add to Allergy-Medication Section.*

Medications

Medication Records

Date _____ Dr. _____ Phone _____

Medication _____ Rx.# _____

Purpose _____

Dosage: _____mg _____ length *(days)*   Other _____

Time:

				Other

Special Instructions *(i.e., taken with food, increase water, etc.)* _____

_____

Side effects (i.e., may cause drowsiness, etc.)_____

_____

Discontinued: Date _____   ❑ Monthly prescription refill

Reason ❑ Completed   ❑ Reaction: *Be sure to add to Allergy-Medication Section.*

Date _____ Dr. _____ Phone _____

Medication _____ Rx.# _____

Purpose _____

Dosage: _____mg _____ length *(days)*   Other _____

Time:

				Other

Special Instructions *(i.e., taken with food, increase water, etc.)* _____

_____

Side effects (i.e., may cause drowsiness, etc.)_____

_____

Discontinued: Date _____   ❑ Monthly prescription refill

Reason ❑ Completed   ❑ Reaction: *Be sure to add to Allergy-Medication Section.*

Date _____ Dr. _____ Phone _____

Medication _____ Rx.# _____

Purpose _____

Dosage: _____mg _____ length *(days)*   Other _____

Time:

				Other

Special Instructions *(i.e., taken with food, increase water, etc.)* _____

_____

Side effects (i.e., may cause drowsiness, etc.)_____

_____

Discontinued: Date _____   ❑ Monthly prescription refill

Reason ❑ Completed   ❑ Reaction: *Be sure to add to Allergy-Medication Section.*

Medications

Medication Records

Date _____ Dr. _____ Phone _____

Medication _____ Rx.# _____

Purpose _____

Dosage: _____mg _____ length *(days)*   Other _____

Time:					Other

Special Instructions *(i.e., taken with food, increase water, etc.)* _____

_____

Side effects (i.e., may cause drowsiness, etc.) _____

_____

Discontinued: Date _____   ❏ Monthly prescription refill

Reason ❏ Completed   ❏ Reaction: *Be sure to add to Allergy-Medication Section.*

Date _____ Dr. _____ Phone _____

Medication _____ Rx.# _____

Purpose _____

Dosage: _____mg _____ length *(days)*   Other _____

Time:					Other

Special Instructions *(i.e., taken with food, increase water, etc.)* _____

_____

Side effects (i.e., may cause drowsiness, etc.) _____

_____

Discontinued: Date _____   ❏ Monthly prescription refill

Reason ❏ Completed   ❏ Reaction: *Be sure to add to Allergy-Medication Section.*

Date _____ Dr. _____ Phone _____

Medication _____ Rx.# _____

Purpose _____

Dosage: _____mg _____ length *(days)*   Other _____

Time:					Other

Special Instructions *(i.e., taken with food, increase water, etc.)* _____

_____

Side effects (i.e., may cause drowsiness, etc.) _____

_____

Discontinued: Date _____   ❏ Monthly prescription refill

Reason ❏ Completed   ❏ Reaction: *Be sure to add to Allergy-Medication Section.*

Medications

Medication Daily Schedule

Medication _____ Date started _____

Time:					Other

Discontinued: Date _____ ❑ Monthly prescription refill Rx # _____

Reason ❑ Completed ❑ Reaction: *Be sure to add to Allergy-Medication Section.*

Medication _____ Date started _____

Time:					Other

Discontinued: Date _____ ❑ Monthly prescription refill Rx # _____

Reason ❑ Completed ❑ Reaction: *Be sure to add to Allergy-Medication Section.*

Medication _____ Date started _____

Time:					Other

Discontinued: Date _____ ❑ Monthly prescription refill Rx # _____

Reason ❑ Completed ❑ Reaction: *Be sure to add to Allergy-Medication Section.*

Medication _____ Date started _____

Time:					Other

Discontinued: Date _____ ❑ Monthly prescription refill Rx # _____

Reason ❑ Completed ❑ Reaction: *Be sure to add to Allergy-Medication Section.*

Medication _____ Date started _____

Time:					Other

Discontinued: Date _____ ❑ Monthly prescription refill Rx # _____

Reason ❑ Completed ❑ Reaction: *Be sure to add to Allergy-Medication Section.*

Medication _____ Date started _____

Time:					Other

Discontinued: Date _____ ❑ Monthly prescription refill Rx # _____

Reason ❑ Completed ❑ Reaction: *Be sure to add to Allergy-Medication Section.*

Medication _____ Date started _____

Time:					Other

Discontinued: Date _____ ❑ Monthly prescription refill Rx # _____

Reason ❑ Completed ❑ Reaction: *Be sure to add to Allergy-Medication Section.*

Medications

Medication Daily Schedule

Medication _____ Date started _____

Time:					Other

Discontinued: Date _____ ❑ Monthly prescription refill Rx # _____

Reason ❑ Completed   ❑ Reaction: *Be sure to add to Allergy-Medication Section.*

Medication _____ Date started _____

Time:					Other

Discontinued: Date _____ ❑ Monthly prescription refill Rx # _____

Reason ❑ Completed   ❑ Reaction: *Be sure to add to Allergy-Medication Section.*

Medication _____ Date started _____

Time:					Other

Discontinued: Date _____ ❑ Monthly prescription refill Rx # _____

Reason ❑ Completed   ❑ Reaction: *Be sure to add to Allergy-Medication Section.*

Medication _____ Date started _____

Time:					Other

Discontinued: Date _____ ❑ Monthly prescription refill Rx # _____

Reason ❑ Completed   ❑ Reaction: *Be sure to add to Allergy-Medication Section.*

Medication _____ Date started _____

Time:					Other

Discontinued: Date _____ ❑ Monthly prescription refill Rx # _____

Reason ❑ Completed   ❑ Reaction: *Be sure to add to Allergy-Medication Section.*

Medication _____ Date started _____

Time:					Other

Discontinued: Date _____ ❑ Monthly prescription refill Rx # _____

Reason ❑ Completed   ❑ Reaction: *Be sure to add to Allergy-Medication Section.*

Medication _____ Date started _____

Time:					Other

Discontinued: Date _____ ❑ Monthly prescription refill Rx # _____

Reason ❑ Completed   ❑ Reaction: *Be sure to add to Allergy-Medication Section.*

Medications

Medication Daily Schedule

Medication _____ Date started _____

Time:					Other

Discontinued: Date _____ ❑ Monthly prescription refill Rx # _____

Reason ❑ Completed   ❑ Reaction: *Be sure to add to Allergy-Medication Section.*

Medication _____ Date started _____

Time: | | | | | Other

Discontinued: Date _____ ❑ Monthly prescription refill Rx # _____

Reason ❑ Completed   ❑ Reaction: *Be sure to add to Allergy-Medication Section.*

Medication _____ Date started _____

Time: | | | | | Other

Discontinued: Date _____ ❑ Monthly prescription refill Rx # _____

Reason ❑ Completed   ❑ Reaction: *Be sure to add to Allergy-Medication Section.*

Medication _____ Date started _____

Time: | | | | | Other

Discontinued: Date _____ ❑ Monthly prescription refill Rx # _____

Reason ❑ Completed   ❑ Reaction: *Be sure to add to Allergy-Medication Section.*

Medication _____ Date started _____

Time: | | | | | Other

Discontinued: Date _____ ❑ Monthly prescription refill Rx # _____

Reason ❑ Completed   ❑ Reaction: *Be sure to add to Allergy-Medication Section.*

Medication _____ Date started _____

Time: | | | | | Other

Discontinued: Date _____ ❑ Monthly prescription refill Rx # _____

Reason ❑ Completed   ❑ Reaction: *Be sure to add to Allergy-Medication Section.*

Medication _____ Date started _____

Time: | | | | | Other

Discontinued: Date _____ ❑ Monthly prescription refill Rx # _____

Reason ❑ Completed   ❑ Reaction: *Be sure to add to Allergy-Medication Section.*

Medications

Medication Daily Schedule

Medication _____ Date started _____

Time: | | | | | Other

Discontinued: Date _____ ❑ Monthly prescription refill Rx # _____
Reason ❑ Completed   ❑ Reaction: *Be sure to add to Allergy-Medication Section.*

Medication _____ Date started _____

Time: | | | | | Other

Discontinued: Date _____ ❑ Monthly prescription refill Rx # _____
Reason ❑ Completed   ❑ Reaction: *Be sure to add to Allergy-Medication Section.*

Medication _____ Date started _____

Time: | | | | | Other

Discontinued: Date _____ ❑ Monthly prescription refill Rx # _____
Reason ❑ Completed   ❑ Reaction: *Be sure to add to Allergy-Medication Section.*

Medication _____ Date started _____

Time: | | | | | Other

Discontinued: Date _____ ❑ Monthly prescription refill Rx # _____
Reason ❑ Completed   ❑ Reaction: *Be sure to add to Allergy-Medication Section.*

Medication _____ Date started _____

Time: | | | | | Other

Discontinued: Date _____ ❑ Monthly prescription refill Rx # _____
Reason ❑ Completed   ❑ Reaction: *Be sure to add to Allergy-Medication Section.*

Medication _____ Date started _____

Time: | | | | | Other

Discontinued: Date _____ ❑ Monthly prescription refill Rx # _____
Reason ❑ Completed   ❑ Reaction: *Be sure to add to Allergy-Medication Section.*

Medication _____ Date started _____

Time: | | | | | Other

Discontinued: Date _____ ❑ Monthly prescription refill Rx # _____
Reason ❑ Completed   ❑ Reaction: *Be sure to add to Allergy-Medication Section.*

Medications

Medication Daily Schedule

Medication _____ Date started _____

Time:					Other

Discontinued: Date _____ ❑ Monthly prescription refill Rx # _____

Reason ❑ Completed   ❑ Reaction: *Be sure to add to Allergy-Medication Section.*

Medication _____ Date started _____

Time:					Other

Discontinued: Date _____ ❑ Monthly prescription refill Rx # _____

Reason ❑ Completed   ❑ Reaction: *Be sure to add to Allergy-Medication Section.*

Medication _____ Date started _____

Time:					Other

Discontinued: Date _____ ❑ Monthly prescription refill Rx # _____

Reason ❑ Completed   ❑ Reaction: *Be sure to add to Allergy-Medication Section.*

Medication _____ Date started _____

Time:					Other

Discontinued: Date _____ ❑ Monthly prescription refill Rx # _____

Reason ❑ Completed   ❑ Reaction: *Be sure to add to Allergy-Medication Section.*

Medication _____ Date started _____

Time:					Other

Discontinued: Date _____ ❑ Monthly prescription refill Rx # _____

Reason ❑ Completed   ❑ Reaction: *Be sure to add to Allergy-Medication Section.*

Medication _____ Date started _____

Time:					Other

Discontinued: Date _____ ❑ Monthly prescription refill Rx # _____

Reason ❑ Completed   ❑ Reaction: *Be sure to add to Allergy-Medication Section.*

Medication _____ Date started _____

Time:					Other

Discontinued: Date _____ ❑ Monthly prescription refill Rx # _____

Reason ❑ Completed   ❑ Reaction: *Be sure to add to Allergy-Medication Section.*

Medications

Medication Daily Schedule

Medication _____ Date started _____

Time: | | | | | Other

Discontinued: Date _____ ❏ Monthly prescription refill Rx # _____

Reason ❏ Completed ❏ Reaction: *Be sure to add to Allergy-Medication Section.*

Medication _____ Date started _____

Time: | | | | | Other

Discontinued: Date _____ ❏ Monthly prescription refill Rx # _____

Reason ❏ Completed ❏ Reaction: *Be sure to add to Allergy-Medication Section.*

Medication _____ Date started _____

Time: | | | | | Other

Discontinued: Date _____ ❏ Monthly prescription refill Rx # _____

Reason ❏ Completed ❏ Reaction: *Be sure to add to Allergy-Medication Section.*

Medication _____ Date started _____

Time: | | | | | Other

Discontinued: Date _____ ❏ Monthly prescription refill Rx # _____

Reason ❏ Completed ❏ Reaction: *Be sure to add to Allergy-Medication Section.*

Medication _____ Date started _____

Time: | | | | | Other

Discontinued: Date _____ ❏ Monthly prescription refill Rx # _____

Reason ❏ Completed ❏ Reaction: *Be sure to add to Allergy-Medication Section.*

Medication _____ Date started _____

Time: | | | | | Other

Discontinued: Date _____ ❏ Monthly prescription refill Rx # _____

Reason ❏ Completed ❏ Reaction: *Be sure to add to Allergy-Medication Section.*

Medication _____ Date started _____

Time: | | | | | Other

Discontinued: Date _____ ❏ Monthly prescription refill Rx # _____

Reason ❏ Completed ❏ Reaction: *Be sure to add to Allergy-Medication Section.*

Medications

Medication Daily Schedule

Medication _____ Date started _____

Time:					Other

Discontinued: Date _____ ❑ Monthly prescription refill Rx # _____

Reason ❑ Completed   ❑ Reaction: *Be sure to add to Allergy-Medication Section.*

Medication _____ Date started _____

Time:					Other

Discontinued: Date _____ ❑ Monthly prescription refill Rx # _____

Reason ❑ Completed   ❑ Reaction: *Be sure to add to Allergy-Medication Section.*

Medication _____ Date started _____

Time:					Other

Discontinued: Date _____ ❑ Monthly prescription refill Rx # _____

Reason ❑ Completed   ❑ Reaction: *Be sure to add to Allergy-Medication Section.*

Medication _____ Date started _____

Time:					Other

Discontinued: Date _____ ❑ Monthly prescription refill Rx # _____

Reason ❑ Completed   ❑ Reaction: *Be sure to add to Allergy-Medication Section.*

Medication _____ Date started _____

Time:					Other

Discontinued: Date _____ ❑ Monthly prescription refill Rx # _____

Reason ❑ Completed   ❑ Reaction: *Be sure to add to Allergy-Medication Section.*

Medication _____ Date started _____

Time:					Other

Discontinued: Date _____ ❑ Monthly prescription refill Rx # _____

Reason ❑ Completed   ❑ Reaction: *Be sure to add to Allergy-Medication Section.*

Medication _____ Date started _____

Time:					Other

Discontinued: Date _____ ❑ Monthly prescription refill Rx # _____

Reason ❑ Completed   ❑ Reaction: *Be sure to add to Allergy-Medication Section.*

Medications

Medication Daily Schedule

Medication _____ Date started _____

Time:					Other

Discontinued: Date _____ ❑ Monthly prescription refill Rx # _____

Reason ❑ Completed   ❑ Reaction: *Be sure to add to Allergy-Medication Section.*

Medication _____ Date started _____

Time:					Other

Discontinued: Date _____ ❑ Monthly prescription refill Rx # _____

Reason ❑ Completed   ❑ Reaction: *Be sure to add to Allergy-Medication Section.*

Medication _____ Date started _____

Time:					Other

Discontinued: Date _____ ❑ Monthly prescription refill Rx # _____

Reason ❑ Completed   ❑ Reaction: *Be sure to add to Allergy-Medication Section.*

Medication _____ Date started _____

Time:					Other

Discontinued: Date _____ ❑ Monthly prescription refill Rx # _____

Reason ❑ Completed   ❑ Reaction: *Be sure to add to Allergy-Medication Section.*

Medication _____ Date started _____

Time:					Other

Discontinued: Date _____ ❑ Monthly prescription refill Rx # _____

Reason ❑ Completed   ❑ Reaction: *Be sure to add to Allergy-Medication Section.*

Medication _____ Date started _____

Time:					Other

Discontinued: Date _____ ❑ Monthly prescription refill Rx # _____

Reason ❑ Completed   ❑ Reaction: *Be sure to add to Allergy-Medication Section.*

Medication _____ Date started _____

Time:					Other

Discontinued: Date _____ ❑ Monthly prescription refill Rx # _____

Reason ❑ Completed   ❑ Reaction: *Be sure to add to Allergy-Medication Section.*

Medications

Medication Daily Schedule

Medication _____ Date started _____

Time: | | | | | Other |
| --- | --- | --- | --- | --- |

Discontinued: Date _____ ❑ Monthly prescription refill Rx # _____

Reason ❑ Completed   ❑ Reaction: *Be sure to add to Allergy-Medication Section.*

Medication _____ Date started _____

Time: | | | | | Other |
| --- | --- | --- | --- | --- |

Discontinued: Date _____ ❑ Monthly prescription refill Rx # _____

Reason ❑ Completed   ❑ Reaction: *Be sure to add to Allergy-Medication Section.*

Medication _____ Date started _____

Time: | | | | | Other |
| --- | --- | --- | --- | --- |

Discontinued: Date _____ ❑ Monthly prescription refill Rx # _____

Reason ❑ Completed   ❑ Reaction: *Be sure to add to Allergy-Medication Section.*

Medication _____ Date started _____

Time: | | | | | Other |
| --- | --- | --- | --- | --- |

Discontinued: Date _____ ❑ Monthly prescription refill Rx # _____

Reason ❑ Completed   ❑ Reaction: *Be sure to add to Allergy-Medication Section.*

Medication _____ Date started _____

Time: | | | | | Other |
| --- | --- | --- | --- | --- |

Discontinued: Date _____ ❑ Monthly prescription refill Rx # _____

Reason ❑ Completed   ❑ Reaction: *Be sure to add to Allergy-Medication Section.*

Medication _____ Date started _____

Time: | | | | | Other |
| --- | --- | --- | --- | --- |

Discontinued: Date _____ ❑ Monthly prescription refill Rx # _____

Reason ❑ Completed   ❑ Reaction: *Be sure to add to Allergy-Medication Section.*

Medication _____ Date started _____

Time: | | | | | Other |
| --- | --- | --- | --- | --- |

Discontinued: Date _____ ❑ Monthly prescription refill Rx # _____

Reason ❑ Completed   ❑ Reaction: *Be sure to add to Allergy-Medication Section.*

Medications

Medication Daily Schedule

Medication _____ Date started _____

Time:

				Other

Discontinued: Date _____ ❑ Monthly prescription refill Rx # _____

Reason ❑ Completed ❑ Reaction: *Be sure to add to Allergy-Medication Section.*

Medication _____ Date started _____

Time:

				Other

Discontinued: Date _____ ❑ Monthly prescription refill Rx # _____

Reason ❑ Completed ❑ Reaction: *Be sure to add to Allergy-Medication Section.*

Medication _____ Date started _____

Time:

				Other

Discontinued: Date _____ ❑ Monthly prescription refill Rx # _____

Reason ❑ Completed ❑ Reaction: *Be sure to add to Allergy-Medication Section.*

Medication _____ Date started _____

Time:

				Other

Discontinued: Date _____ ❑ Monthly prescription refill Rx # _____

Reason ❑ Completed ❑ Reaction: *Be sure to add to Allergy-Medication Section.*

Medication _____ Date started _____

Time:

				Other

Discontinued: Date _____ ❑ Monthly prescription refill Rx # _____

Reason ❑ Completed ❑ Reaction: *Be sure to add to Allergy-Medication Section.*

Medication _____ Date started _____

Time:

				Other

Discontinued: Date _____ ❑ Monthly prescription refill Rx # _____

Reason ❑ Completed ❑ Reaction: *Be sure to add to Allergy-Medication Section.*

Medication _____ Date started _____

Time:

				Other

Discontinued: Date _____ ❑ Monthly prescription refill Rx # _____

Reason ❑ Completed ❑ Reaction: *Be sure to add to Allergy-Medication Section.*

Medications

Alerts — Concerns

Alerts — Concerns: Write any health and/or medical concerns that occur, or areas that need to be continually observed.

Notes

Alerts – Concerns

Date _____ Dr. / Other _____

Condition / Diagnosis _____

_____

❑ Lab ❑ X-ray ❑ Other Tests _____

NEXT APPOINTMENT: Date _____ Time _____

Describe _____

_____

_____

Date _____ Dr. / Other _____

Condition / Diagnosis _____

_____

❑ Lab ❑ X-ray ❑ Other Tests _____

NEXT APPOINTMENT: Date _____ Time _____

Describe _____

_____

_____

Date _____ Dr. / Other _____

Condition / Diagnosis _____

_____

❑ Lab ❑ X-ray ❑ Other Tests _____

NEXT APPOINTMENT: Date _____ Time _____

Describe _____

_____

_____

Alerts - Concerns

Alerts – Concerns

Date _____ Dr. / Other _____

Condition / Diagnosis _____

_____

❑ Lab   ❑ X-ray   ❑ Other Tests _____

NEXT APPOINTMENT: Date _____ Time _____

Describe _____

_____

_____

_____

Date _____ Dr. / Other _____

Condition / Diagnosis _____

_____

❑ Lab   ❑ X-ray   ❑ Other Tests _____

NEXT APPOINTMENT: Date _____ Time _____

Describe _____

_____

_____

_____

Date _____ Dr. / Other _____

Condition / Diagnosis _____

_____

❑ Lab   ❑ X-ray   ❑ Other Tests _____

NEXT APPOINTMENT: Date _____ Time _____

Describe _____

_____

_____

_____

Alerts - Concerns

Alerts – Concerns

Date _____ Dr. / Other _____

Condition / Diagnosis _____

_____

❑ Lab ❑ X-ray ❑ Other Tests _____

NEXT APPOINTMENT: Date _____ Time _____

Describe _____

_____

_____

Date _____ Dr. / Other _____

Condition / Diagnosis _____

_____

❑ Lab ❑ X-ray ❑ Other Tests _____

NEXT APPOINTMENT: Date _____ Time _____

Describe _____

_____

_____

Date _____ Dr. / Other _____

Condition / Diagnosis _____

_____

❑ Lab ❑ X-ray ❑ Other Tests _____

NEXT APPOINTMENT: Date _____ Time _____

Describe _____

_____

_____

Alerts – Concerns

Date _____ Dr. / Other _____

Condition / Diagnosis _____

_____

❑ Lab ❑ X-ray ❑ Other Tests _____

NEXT APPOINTMENT: Date _____ Time _____

Describe _____

_____

_____

Date _____ Dr. / Other _____

Condition / Diagnosis _____

_____

❑ Lab ❑ X-ray ❑ Other Tests _____

NEXT APPOINTMENT: Date _____ Time _____

Describe _____

_____

_____

Date _____ Dr. / Other _____

Condition / Diagnosis _____

_____

❑ Lab ❑ X-ray ❑ Other Tests _____

NEXT APPOINTMENT: Date _____ Time _____

Describe _____

_____

_____

Alerts - Concerns

Alerts – Concerns

Date _____ Dr. / Other _____

Condition / Diagnosis _____

_____

❏ Lab ❏ X-ray ❏ Other Tests _____

NEXT APPOINTMENT: Date _____ Time _____

Describe _____

_____

_____

Date _____ Dr. / Other _____

Condition / Diagnosis _____

_____

❏ Lab ❏ X-ray ❏ Other Tests _____

NEXT APPOINTMENT: Date _____ Time _____

Describe _____

_____

_____

Date _____ Dr. / Other _____

Condition / Diagnosis _____

_____

❏ Lab ❏ X-ray ❏ Other Tests _____

NEXT APPOINTMENT: Date _____ Time _____

Describe _____

_____

_____

Alerts – Concerns

Date _____ Dr. / Other _____

Condition / Diagnosis _____

_____

❏ Lab   ❏ X-ray   ❏ Other Tests _____

NEXT APPOINTMENT: Date _____ Time _____

Describe _____

_____

_____

Date _____ Dr. / Other _____

Condition / Diagnosis _____

_____

❏ Lab   ❏ X-ray   ❏ Other Tests _____

NEXT APPOINTMENT: Date _____ Time _____

Describe _____

_____

_____

Date _____ Dr. / Other _____

Condition / Diagnosis _____

_____

❏ Lab   ❏ X-ray   ❏ Other Tests _____

NEXT APPOINTMENT: Date _____ Time _____

Describe _____

_____

_____

Alerts - Concerns

Hospitalizations * Surgeries * Procedures Log
Hospitalizations * Surgeries * Procedures Records

Hospitalizations * Surgeries * Procedures: You, the physician, or the dentist can summarize the procedure, complications, and any notes in this area. Ask for a copy of his/her notes for your file/binder.

Notes

Hospitalizations * Surgeries * Procedures Log

Place a (✓) in the appropriate category.

DATE	TYPE	HOSPITALIZATION	SURGERY	PROCEDURE	COMMENTS

Hospitalizations * Surgeries * Procedures Log

Place a (✓) in the appropriate category.

DATE	TYPE	HOSPITALIZATION	SURGERY	PROCEDURE	COMMENTS

Hospitalizations
Surgeries * Procedures

Hospitalizations * Surgeries * Procedures Log

Place a (✓) in the appropriate category.

DATE	TYPE	HOSPITALIZATION	SURGERY	PROCEDURE	COMMENTS

Hospitalizations * Surgeries * Procedures Log

Place a (✓) in the appropriate category.

DATE	TYPE	HOSPITALIZATION	SURGERY	PROCEDURE	COMMENTS

**Hospitalizations
Surgeries * Procedures**

Hospitalizations * Surgeries * Procedures Records

❏ **HOSPITALIZATION**   ❏ **SURGERY**   ❏ **PROCEDURE**

(Best to use a separate page for each category.)

Date _____

Medical Facility _____

City _____ State _____

Phone_____ Other_____

Temperature _____Blood pressure _____ Pulse _____

Glucose _____Other _____

Blood Test _____

Anesthesia _____ Dr. _____

Reaction ❏ No ❏ Yes _____

_____

_____

Counteraction _____

_____

_____

Dr. _____ Dr. _____

Procedure_____

_____

_____

Summary _____

_____

_____

Complications _____

_____

Length of Stay_____

Discharge / Care Instructions. ❏ *See hospital discharge instructions.*

Add a separate page if you need to write more detail.

Hospitalizations * Surgeries * Procedures Records

❏ **HOSPITALIZATION**   ❏ **SURGERY**   ❏ **PROCEDURE**
(Best to use a separate page for each category.)

Date _____

Medical Facility _____

City _____ State _____

Phone _____ Other _____

Temperature _____ Blood pressure _____ Pulse _____

Glucose _____ Other _____

Blood Test _____

Anesthesia _____ Dr. _____

Reaction ❏ No ❏ Yes _____

_____

_____

Counteraction _____

_____

_____

Dr. _____ Dr. _____

Procedure _____

_____

_____

Summary _____

_____

_____

Complications _____

_____

Length of Stay _____

Discharge / Care Instructions. ❏ *See hospital discharge instructions.*

Add a separate page if you need to write more detail.

Hospitalizations * Surgeries * Procedures Records

❏ **HOSPITALIZATION**   ❏ **SURGERY**   ❏ **PROCEDURE**

(Best to use a separate page for each category.)

Date _____

Medical Facility _____

City _____ State _____

Phone _____ Other _____

Temperature _____ Blood pressure _____ Pulse _____

Glucose _____ Other _____

Blood Test _____

Anesthesia _____ Dr. _____

Reaction ❏ No ❏ Yes _____

_____

_____

Counteraction _____

_____

_____

Dr. _____ Dr. _____

Procedure _____

_____

_____

Summary _____

_____

_____

Complications _____

_____

Length of Stay _____

Discharge / Care Instructions. ❏ *See hospital discharge instructions.*

Add a separate page if you need to write more detail.

Hospitalizations * Surgeries * Procedures Records

❏ **HOSPITALIZATION**   ❏ **SURGERY**   ❏ **PROCEDURE**

(Best to use a separate page for each category.)

Date _____

Medical Facility _____

City _____ State _____

Phone _____ Other _____

Temperature _____ Blood pressure _____ Pulse _____

Glucose _____ Other _____

Blood Test _____

Anesthesia _____ Dr. _____

Reaction ❏ No ❏ Yes _____

_____

_____

Counteraction _____

_____

_____

Dr. _____ Dr. _____

Procedure _____

_____

_____

Summary _____

_____

_____

Complications _____

_____

Length of Stay _____

Discharge / Care Instructions. ❏ *See hospital discharge instructions.*

Add a separate page if you need to write more detail.

Hospitalizations * Surgeries * Procedures Records

❏ **HOSPITALIZATION**   ❏ **SURGERY**   ❏ **PROCEDURE**
(Best to use a separate page for each category.)

Date _____

Medical Facility _____

City _____ State _____

Phone_____ Other _____

Temperature _____ Blood pressure _____ Pulse _____

Glucose _____ Other _____

Blood Test _____

Anesthesia _____ Dr. _____

Reaction ❏ No ❏ Yes _____

_____

_____

Counteraction _____

_____

_____

Dr. _____ Dr. _____

Procedure_____

_____

_____

Summary _____

_____

_____

Complications _____

_____

Length of Stay_____

Discharge / Care Instructions. ❏ *See hospital discharge instructions.*

Add a separate page if you need to write more detail.

Hospitalizations * Surgeries * Procedures Records

❏ **HOSPITALIZATION**   ❏ **SURGERY**   ❏ **PROCEDURE**

(Best to use a separate page for each category.)

Date _____

Medical Facility _____

City _____ State _____

Phone_____ Other_____

Temperature_____Blood pressure_____ Pulse _____

Glucose _____Other _____

Blood Test _____

Anesthesia _____ Dr. _____

Reaction ❏ No ❏ Yes _____

_____

_____

Counteraction _____

_____

_____

Dr. _____ Dr. _____

Procedure_____

_____

_____

Summary _____

_____

_____

Complications _____

_____

Length of Stay_____

Discharge / Care Instructions. ❏ *See hospital discharge instructions.*

Add a separate page if you need to write more detail.

Hospitalizations * Surgeries * Procedures Records

❏ **HOSPITALIZATION**   ❏ **SURGERY**   ❏ **PROCEDURE**
(Best to use a separate page for each category.)

Date _____

Medical Facility _____

City _____ State _____

Phone_____ Other _____

Temperature_____Blood pressure _____ Pulse _____

Glucose _____Other _____

Blood Test _____

Anesthesia _____ Dr. _____

Reaction ❏ No ❏ Yes _____

_____

_____

Counteraction _____

_____

_____

Dr. _____ Dr. _____

Procedure_____

_____

_____

Summary _____

_____

_____

Complications _____

_____

Length of Stay_____

Discharge / Care Instructions. ❏ *See hospital discharge instructions.*

Add a separate page if you need to write more detail.

Hospitalizations * Surgeries * Procedures Records

❏ **HOSPITALIZATION**   ❏ **SURGERY**   ❏ **PROCEDURE**
(Best to use a separate page for each category.)

Date _____

Medical Facility _____

City _____ State _____

Phone _____ Other _____

Temperature _____ Blood pressure _____ Pulse _____

Glucose _____ Other _____

Blood Test _____

Anesthesia _____ Dr. _____

Reaction ❏ No ❏ Yes _____

_____

_____

Counteraction _____

_____

_____

Dr. _____ Dr. _____

Procedure _____

_____

_____

Summary _____

_____

_____

Complications _____

_____

Length of Stay _____

Discharge / Care Instructions. ❏ *See hospital discharge instructions.*

Add a separate page if you need to write more detail.

Hospitalizations * Surgeries * Procedures Records

❑ **HOSPITALIZATION**   ❑ **SURGERY**   ❑ **PROCEDURE**

(Best to use a separate page for each category.)

Date _____

Medical Facility _____

City _____ State _____

Phone _____ Other _____

Temperature _____ Blood pressure _____ Pulse _____

Glucose _____ Other _____

Blood Test _____

Anesthesia _____ Dr. _____

Reaction ❑ No ❑ Yes _____

_____

_____

Counteraction _____

_____

_____

Dr. _____ Dr. _____

Procedure _____

_____

_____

Summary _____

_____

_____

Complications _____

_____

Length of Stay _____

Discharge / Care Instructions. ❑ *See hospital discharge instructions.*

Add a separate page if you need to write more detail.

Hospitalizations * Surgeries * Procedures Records

❑ **HOSPITALIZATION**   ❑ **SURGERY**   ❑ **PROCEDURE**
(Best to use a separate page for each category.)

Date _____

Medical Facility _____

City _____ State _____

Phone _____ Other _____

Temperature _____ Blood pressure _____ Pulse _____

Glucose _____ Other _____

Blood Test _____

Anesthesia _____ Dr. _____

Reaction ❑ No ❑ Yes _____

_____

_____

Counteraction _____

_____

_____

Dr. _____ Dr. _____

Procedure _____

_____

_____

Summary _____

_____

_____

Complications _____

_____

Length of Stay _____

Discharge / Care Instructions. ❑ *See hospital discharge instructions.*

Add a separate page if you need to write more detail.

Medical
Appointment Records

Medical Appointments * Doctor Visits: Write the reason for the visit (routine, emergency, etc). This is especially helpful to keep abreast of what has occurred, and for a continuum of health. You can have the doctor summarize the procedure, complications, and any notes in this area. If you feel it is needed, ask the doctor for a copy of his/her notes for your file/binder.

Notes

Medical
Appointment Records

☐ **DOCTOR VISITS**   ☐ **OTHER SERVICES**   ☐ **THERAPISTS**

(Best to use a separate page for each category.)   Year _____

Date _____ Dr. / Other _____

Purpose _____

_____

Temperature _____ Blood Pressure _____ Pulse _____

Glucose _____ Other _____ Weight _____

Blood Test _____

☐ Lab   ☐ X-ray   ☐ Other Tests _____

☐ Special Referral   Dr. / Other _____

Phone (   ) _____   ☐ Referral Slip   ☐ X-ray Copy

Purpose _____

_____

_____

Next Appointment: Date _____ Time _____

☐ Request copy of Dr.'s report sent to Home and ☐ Other _____

Visit Summary _____

_____

_____

_____

QUESTIONS - CONCERNS
(It is always helpful to have your list ready before your meeting.)

Date _____ Dr. / Other _____

_____

_____

_____

_____

_____

_____

Medical
Appointment Records

❑ **DOCTOR VISITS**   ❑ **OTHER SERVICES**   ❑ **THERAPISTS**

(Best to use a separate page for each category.)   Year _____

Date _____Dr. / Other _____

Purpose _____

_____

Temperature _____Blood Pressure _____Pulse _____

Glucose _____Other _____Weight _____

Blood Test _____

❑ Lab   ❑ X-ray   ❑ Other Tests _____

❑ Special Referral   Dr. / Other _____

Phone (   ) _____   ❑ Referral Slip   ❑ X-ray Copy

Purpose _____

_____

_____

Next Appointment: Date _____Time_____

❑ Request copy of Dr.'s report sent to Home and ❑ Other_____

Visit Summary _____

_____

_____

QUESTIONS - CONCERNS
(It is always helpful to have your list ready before your meeting.)

Date _____Dr. / Other _____

_____

_____

_____

_____

_____

_____

Medical
Appointment Records

☐ **DOCTOR VISITS**　　☐ **OTHER SERVICES**　　☐ **THERAPISTS**

(Best to use a separate page for each category.)　　　Year _____

Date _____Dr. / Other _____

Purpose _____
_____

Temperature_____Blood Pressure_____Pulse _____

Glucose _____Other _____Weight _____

Blood Test _____

☐ Lab　☐ X-ray　☐ Other Tests _____

☐ Special Referral　Dr. / Other _____

Phone (　　)_____　☐ Referral Slip　☐ X-ray Copy

Purpose_____
_____
_____

Next Appointment:　Date _____Time_____

☐ Request copy of Dr.'s report sent to Home and ☐ Other_____

Visit Summary _____
_____
_____

QUESTIONS - CONCERNS
(It is always helpful to have your list ready before your meeting.)

Date _____Dr. / Other _____
_____
_____
_____
_____
_____
_____

Medical
Appointment Records

❑ **DOCTOR VISITS**   ❑ **OTHER SERVICES**   ❑ **THERAPISTS**

(Best to use a separate page for each category.)   Year _____

Date _____Dr. / Other _____

Purpose _____

_____

Temperature_____Blood Pressure_____Pulse _____

Glucose _____Other _____Weight _____

Blood Test _____

❑ Lab   ❑ X-ray   ❑ Other Tests _____

❑ Special Referral   Dr. / Other _____

Phone (   )_____   ❑ Referral Slip   ❑ X-ray Copy

Purpose_____

_____

_____

Next Appointment: Date _____Time_____

❑ Request copy of Dr.'s report sent to Home and ❑ Other_____

Visit Summary _____

_____

_____

QUESTIONS - CONCERNS
(It is always helpful to have your list ready before your meeting.)

Date _____Dr. / Other _____

_____

_____

_____

_____

_____

_____

Medical
Appointment Records

❏ **DOCTOR VISITS**   ❏ **OTHER SERVICES**   ❏ **THERAPISTS**

(Best to use a separate page for each category.)   Year _____

Date _____Dr. / Other _____

Purpose _____

_____

Temperature_____Blood Pressure_____Pulse _____

Glucose _____Other _____Weight _____

Blood Test _____

❏ Lab   ❏ X-ray   ❏ Other Tests _____

❏ Special Referral   Dr. / Other _____

Phone (   )_____   ❏ Referral Slip   ❏ X-ray Copy

Purpose_____

_____

_____

Next Appointment: Date _____Time_____

❏ Request copy of Dr.'s report sent to Home and ❏ Other_____

Visit Summary _____

_____

_____

QUESTIONS - CONCERNS
(It is always helpful to have your list ready before your meeting.)

Date _____Dr. / Other _____

_____

_____

_____

_____

_____

_____

Medical
Appointment Records

❑ **DOCTOR VISITS** ❑ **OTHER SERVICES** ❑ **THERAPISTS**

(Best to use a separate page for each category.) Year _____

Date _____ Dr. / Other _____

Purpose _____

_____

Temperature _____ Blood Pressure _____ Pulse _____

Glucose _____ Other _____ Weight _____

Blood Test _____

❑ Lab ❑ X-ray ❑ Other Tests _____

❑ Special Referral Dr. / Other _____

Phone (   ) _____ ❑ Referral Slip ❑ X-ray Copy

Purpose _____

_____

_____

Next Appointment: Date _____ Time_____

❑ Request copy of Dr.'s report sent to Home and ❑ Other_____

Visit Summary _____

_____

_____

QUESTIONS - CONCERNS
(It is always helpful to have your list ready before your meeting.)

Date _____ Dr. / Other _____

_____

_____

_____

_____

_____

_____

Medical
Appointment Records

❏ **DOCTOR VISITS**　　❏ **OTHER SERVICES**　　❏ **THERAPISTS**

(Best to use a separate page for each category.)　　　Year _____

Date _____ Dr. / Other _____

Purpose _____

_____

Temperature _____ Blood Pressure _____ Pulse _____

Glucose _____ Other _____ Weight _____

Blood Test _____

❏ Lab　❏ X-ray　❏ Other Tests _____

❏ Special Referral　Dr. / Other _____

Phone (   ) _____　❏ Referral Slip　❏ X-ray Copy

Purpose _____

_____

_____

Next Appointment:　Date _____ Time _____

❏ Request copy of Dr.'s report sent to Home and ❏ Other _____

Visit Summary _____

_____

_____

_____

QUESTIONS - CONCERNS
(It is always helpful to have your list ready before your meeting.)

Date _____ Dr. / Other _____

_____

_____

_____

_____

_____

_____

Medical
Appointment Records

❏ **DOCTOR VISITS**   ❏ **OTHER SERVICES**   ❏ **THERAPISTS**

(Best to use a separate page for each category.)   Year _____

Date _____Dr. / Other _____

Purpose _____

_____

Temperature _____Blood Pressure _____Pulse _____

Glucose _____Other _____Weight _____

Blood Test _____

❏ Lab   ❏ X-ray   ❏ Other Tests _____

❏ Special Referral   Dr. / Other _____

Phone (   )_____   ❏ Referral Slip   ❏ X-ray Copy

Purpose_____

_____

_____

Next Appointment: Date _____Time_____

❏ Request copy of Dr.'s report sent to Home and ❏ Other_____

Visit Summary _____

_____

_____

QUESTIONS - CONCERNS
(It is always helpful to have your list ready before your meeting.)

Date _____Dr. / Other _____

_____

_____

_____

_____

_____

_____

Medical
Appointment Records

❑ **DOCTOR VISITS**   ❑ **OTHER SERVICES**   ❑ **THERAPISTS**

(Best to use a separate page for each category.)   Year _____

Date _____Dr. / Other _____

Purpose _____

_____

Temperature_____Blood Pressure_____Pulse _____

Glucose _____Other _____Weight _____

Blood Test _____

❑ Lab   ❑ X-ray   ❑ Other Tests _____

❑ Special Referral   Dr. / Other _____

Phone (   )_____   ❑ Referral Slip   ❑ X-ray Copy

Purpose_____

_____

_____

Next Appointment: Date _____Time_____

❑ Request copy of Dr.'s report sent to Home and ❑ Other_____

Visit Summary _____

_____

_____

_____

QUESTIONS - CONCERNS
(It is always helpful to have your list ready before your meeting.)

Date _____Dr. / Other _____

_____

_____

_____

_____

_____

_____

Medical
Appointment Records

❏ **DOCTOR VISITS**   ❏ **OTHER SERVICES**   ❏ **THERAPISTS**

(Best to use a separate page for each category.)   Year _____

Date _____Dr. / Other _____

Purpose _____

_____

Temperature_____Blood Pressure_____Pulse _____

Glucose _____Other _____Weight _____

Blood Test _____

❏ Lab   ❏ X-ray   ❏ Other Tests _____

❏ Special Referral   Dr. / Other _____

Phone (   )_____   ❏ Referral Slip   ❏ X-ray Copy

Purpose_____

_____

_____

Next Appointment: Date _____Time_____

❏ Request copy of Dr.'s report sent to Home and ❏ Other_____

Visit Summary _____

_____

_____

QUESTIONS - CONCERNS
(It is always helpful to have your list ready before your meeting.)

Date _____Dr. / Other _____

_____

_____

_____

_____

_____

_____

Medical
Appointment Records

❏ **DOCTOR VISITS**　　❏ **OTHER SERVICES**　　❏ **THERAPISTS**

(Best to use a separate page for each category.)　　Year _____

Date _____Dr. / Other _____

Purpose _____

_____

Temperature_____Blood Pressure_____Pulse _____

Glucose _____Other _____Weight _____

Blood Test _____

❏ Lab　❏ X-ray　❏ Other Tests_____

❏ Special Referral　Dr. / Other _____

Phone (　　　) _____　❏ Referral Slip　❏ X-ray Copy

Purpose_____

_____

_____

Next Appointment:　Date _____Time_____

❏ Request copy of Dr.'s report sent to Home and ❏ Other_____

Visit Summary _____

_____

_____

QUESTIONS - CONCERNS
(It is always helpful to have your list ready before your meeting.)

Date _____Dr. / Other _____

_____

_____

_____

_____

_____

_____

Medical
Appointment Records

❑ **DOCTOR VISITS**   ❑ **OTHER SERVICES**   ❑ **THERAPISTS**

(Best to use a separate page for each category.)   Year _____

Date _____Dr. / Other _____

Purpose _____

_____

Temperature_____Blood Pressure_____Pulse _____

Glucose _____Other _____Weight _____

Blood Test _____

❑ Lab   ❑ X-ray   ❑ Other Tests_____

❑ Special Referral   Dr. / Other _____

Phone (   )_____   ❑ Referral Slip   ❑ X-ray Copy

Purpose_____

_____

_____

Next Appointment: Date _____Time_____

❑ Request copy of Dr.'s report sent to Home and ❑ Other_____

Visit Summary _____

_____

_____

QUESTIONS - CONCERNS
(It is always helpful to have your list ready before your meeting.)

Date _____Dr. / Other _____

_____

_____

_____

_____

_____

_____

Medical
Appointment Records

❏ **DOCTOR VISITS**   ❏ **OTHER SERVICES**   ❏ **THERAPISTS**

(Best to use a separate page for each category.)   Year _____

Date _____ Dr. / Other _____

Purpose _____

_____

Temperature _____ Blood Pressure _____ Pulse _____

Glucose _____ Other _____ Weight _____

Blood Test _____

❏ Lab   ❏ X-ray   ❏ Other Tests _____

❏ Special Referral   Dr. / Other _____

Phone (   ) _____   ❏ Referral Slip   ❏ X-ray Copy

Purpose _____

_____

_____

Next Appointment: Date _____ Time _____

❏ Request copy of Dr.'s report sent to Home and ❏ Other _____

Visit Summary _____

_____

_____

_____

QUESTIONS - CONCERNS
(It is always helpful to have your list ready before your meeting.)

Date _____ Dr. / Other _____

_____

_____

_____

_____

_____

_____

Medical
Appointment Records

❑ **DOCTOR VISITS**　　❑ **OTHER SERVICES**　　❑ **THERAPISTS**

(Best to use a separate page for each category.)　　　　Year _____

Date _____Dr. / Other _____

Purpose _____

_____

Temperature _____Blood Pressure _____Pulse _____

Glucose _____Other _____Weight _____

Blood Test _____

❑ Lab　 ❑ X-ray　 ❑ Other Tests _____

❑ Special Referral　 Dr. / Other _____

Phone (　　　) _____　 ❑ Referral Slip　 ❑ X-ray Copy

Purpose_____

_____

_____

Next Appointment:　 Date _____Time_____

❑ Request copy of Dr.'s report sent to Home and ❑ Other_____

Visit Summary _____

_____

_____

_____

QUESTIONS - CONCERNS
(It is always helpful to have your list ready before your meeting.)

Date _____Dr. / Other _____

_____

_____

_____

_____

_____

_____

Medical
Appointment Records

❑ **DOCTOR VISITS**　　❑ **OTHER SERVICES**　　❑ **THERAPISTS**

(Best to use a separate page for each category.)　　　　Year _____

Date _____Dr. / Other _____

Purpose _____

_____

Temperature _____Blood Pressure _____Pulse _____

Glucose _____Other _____Weight _____

Blood Test _____

❑ Lab　❑ X-ray　❑ Other Tests _____

❑ Special Referral　Dr. / Other _____

Phone (　　)_____　❑ Referral Slip　❑ X-ray Copy

Purpose_____

_____

_____

Next Appointment:　Date _____Time_____

❑ Request copy of Dr.'s report sent to Home and ❑ Other_____

Visit Summary _____

_____

_____

_____

QUESTIONS - CONCERNS
(It is always helpful to have your list ready before your meeting.)

Date _____Dr. / Other _____

_____

_____

_____

_____

_____

_____

Medical
Appointment Records

❏ **DOCTOR VISITS**   ❏ **OTHER SERVICES**   ❏ **THERAPISTS**

(Best to use a separate page for each category.)   Year _____

Date _____Dr. / Other _____

Purpose _____

_____

Temperature_____Blood Pressure_____Pulse _____

Glucose _____Other _____Weight _____

Blood Test _____

❏ Lab   ❏ X-ray   ❏ Other Tests _____

❏ Special Referral   Dr. / Other _____

Phone (   )_____   ❏ Referral Slip   ❏ X-ray Copy

Purpose_____

_____

_____

Next Appointment: Date _____Time_____

❏ Request copy of Dr.'s report sent to Home and ❏ Other_____

Visit Summary _____

_____

_____

QUESTIONS - CONCERNS
(It is always helpful to have your list ready before your meeting.)

Date _____Dr. / Other _____

_____

_____

_____

_____

_____

_____

Medical
Appointment Records

❏ **DOCTOR VISITS**   ❏ **OTHER SERVICES**   ❏ **THERAPISTS**

(Best to use a separate page for each category.)   Year _____

Date _____Dr. / Other _____

Purpose _____

_____

Temperature_____Blood Pressure_____Pulse _____

Glucose _____Other _____Weight _____

Blood Test _____

❏ Lab   ❏ X-ray   ❏ Other Tests_____

❏ Special Referral   Dr. / Other _____

Phone (   )_____   ❏ Referral Slip   ❏ X-ray Copy

Purpose_____

_____

_____

Next Appointment: Date _____Time_____

❏ Request copy of Dr.'s report sent to Home and ❏ Other_____

Visit Summary _____

_____

_____

QUESTIONS - CONCERNS
(It is always helpful to have your list ready before your meeting.)

Date _____Dr. / Other _____

_____

_____

_____

_____

_____

_____

105

Medical
Appointment Records

❏ **DOCTOR VISITS**   ❏ **OTHER SERVICES**   ❏ **THERAPISTS**

(Best to use a separate page for each category.)   Year _____

Date _____Dr. / Other _____

Purpose _____

_____

Temperature_____Blood Pressure_____Pulse _____

Glucose _____Other _____Weight _____

Blood Test _____

❏ Lab   ❏ X-ray   ❏ Other Tests _____

❏ Special Referral   Dr. / Other _____

Phone (   )_____   ❏ Referral Slip   ❏ X-ray Copy

Purpose_____

_____

_____

Next Appointment: Date _____Time_____

❏ Request copy of Dr.'s report sent to Home and ❏ Other_____

Visit Summary _____

_____

_____

QUESTIONS - CONCERNS
(It is always helpful to have your list ready before your meeting.)

Date _____Dr. / Other _____

_____

_____

_____

_____

_____

_____

Medical
Appointment Records

❏ **DOCTOR VISITS**   ❏ **OTHER SERVICES**   ❏ **THERAPISTS**

(Best to use a separate page for each category.)   Year _____

Date _____Dr. / Other _____

Purpose _____

_____

Temperature_____Blood Pressure_____Pulse _____

Glucose _____Other _____Weight _____

Blood Test _____

❏ Lab   ❏ X-ray   ❏ Other Tests _____

❏ Special Referral   Dr. / Other _____

Phone (   )_____   ❏ Referral Slip   ❏ X-ray Copy

Purpose_____

_____

_____

Next Appointment: Date _____Time_____

❏ Request copy of Dr.'s report sent to Home and ❏ Other_____

Visit Summary _____

_____

_____

_____

QUESTIONS - CONCERNS
(It is always helpful to have your list ready before your meeting.)

Date _____Dr. / Other _____

_____

_____

_____

_____

_____

_____

Medical
Appointment Records

❏ **DOCTOR VISITS**   ❏ **OTHER SERVICES**   ❏ **THERAPISTS**
(Best to use a separate page for each category.)   Year _____

Date _____Dr. / Other _____

Purpose _____

_____

Temperature _____Blood Pressure _____Pulse _____

Glucose _____Other _____Weight _____

Blood Test _____

❏ Lab   ❏ X-ray   ❏ Other Tests _____

❏ Special Referral   Dr. / Other _____

Phone (   ) _____   ❏ Referral Slip   ❏ X-ray Copy

Purpose _____

_____

_____

Next Appointment: Date _____Time _____

❏ Request copy of Dr.'s report sent to Home and ❏ Other _____

Visit Summary _____

_____

_____

QUESTIONS - CONCERNS
(It is always helpful to have your list ready before your meeting.)

Date _____Dr. / Other _____

_____

_____

_____

_____

_____

Medical
Appointment Records

❏ **DOCTOR VISITS**   ❏ **OTHER SERVICES**   ❏ **THERAPISTS**

(Best to use a separate page for each category.)   Year _____

Date _____Dr. / Other _____

Purpose _____

_____

Temperature_____Blood Pressure_____Pulse _____

Glucose _____Other _____Weight _____

Blood Test _____

❏ Lab   ❏ X-ray   ❏ Other Tests _____

❏ Special Referral   Dr. / Other _____

Phone (   )_____   ❏ Referral Slip   ❏ X-ray Copy

Purpose_____

_____

_____

Next Appointment: Date _____Time_____

❏ Request copy of Dr.'s report sent to Home and ❏ Other_____

Visit Summary _____

_____

_____

_____

QUESTIONS - CONCERNS
(It is always helpful to have your list ready before your meeting.)

Date _____Dr. / Other _____

_____

_____

_____

_____

_____

_____

_____

Medical
Appointment Records

❑ **DOCTOR VISITS**   ❑ **OTHER SERVICES**   ❑ **THERAPISTS**

(Best to use a separate page for each category.)   Year _____

Date _____Dr. / Other _____

Purpose _____

_____

Temperature_____Blood Pressure_____Pulse _____

Glucose _____Other _____Weight _____

Blood Test _____

❑ Lab   ❑ X-ray   ❑ Other Tests _____

❑ Special Referral   Dr. / Other _____

Phone (   )_____   ❑ Referral Slip   ❑ X-ray Copy

Purpose_____

_____

_____

Next Appointment: Date _____Time_____

❑ Request copy of Dr.'s report sent to Home and ❑ Other_____

Visit Summary _____

_____

_____

QUESTIONS - CONCERNS
(It is always helpful to have your list ready before your meeting.)

Date _____Dr. / Other _____

_____

_____

_____

_____

_____

_____

Medical
Appointment Records

❏ **DOCTOR VISITS**   ❏ **OTHER SERVICES**   ❏ **THERAPISTS**

(Best to use a separate page for each category.)   Year _____

Date _____Dr. / Other _____

Purpose _____

_____

Temperature_____Blood Pressure_____Pulse _____

Glucose _____Other _____Weight _____

Blood Test _____

❏ Lab   ❏ X-ray   ❏ Other Tests_____

❏ Special Referral   Dr. / Other _____

Phone (   )_____   ❏ Referral Slip   ❏ X-ray Copy

Purpose_____

_____

_____

Next Appointment: Date _____Time_____

❏ Request copy of Dr.'s report sent to Home and ❏ Other_____

Visit Summary _____

_____

_____

QUESTIONS - CONCERNS
(It is always helpful to have your list ready before your meeting.)

Date _____Dr. / Other _____

_____

_____

_____

_____

_____

_____

Medical
Appointment Records

❏ **DOCTOR VISITS**   ❏ **OTHER SERVICES**   ❏ **THERAPISTS**

(Best to use a separate page for each category.)   Year _____

Date _____ Dr. / Other _____

Purpose _____

_____

Temperature _____ Blood Pressure _____ Pulse _____

Glucose _____ Other _____ Weight _____

Blood Test _____

❏ Lab   ❏ X-ray   ❏ Other Tests _____

❏ Special Referral   Dr. / Other _____

Phone (   ) _____   ❏ Referral Slip   ❏ X-ray Copy

Purpose _____

_____

_____

Next Appointment: Date _____ Time _____

❏ Request copy of Dr.'s report sent to Home and ❏ Other _____

Visit Summary _____

_____

_____

QUESTIONS - CONCERNS
(It is always helpful to have your list ready before your meeting.)

Date _____ Dr. / Other _____

_____

_____

_____

_____

_____

_____

Medical
Appointment Records

☐ **DOCTOR VISITS**   ☐ **OTHER SERVICES**   ☐ **THERAPISTS**

(Best to use a separate page for each category.)   Year _____

Date _____ Dr. / Other _____

Purpose _____

_____

Temperature _____ Blood Pressure _____ Pulse _____

Glucose _____ Other _____ Weight _____

Blood Test _____

☐ Lab   ☐ X-ray   ☐ Other Tests _____

☐ Special Referral   Dr. / Other _____

Phone (_____) _____   ☐ Referral Slip   ☐ X-ray Copy

Purpose_____

_____

_____

Next Appointment: Date _____ Time_____

☐ Request copy of Dr.'s report sent to Home and ☐ Other_____

Visit Summary _____

_____

_____

QUESTIONS - CONCERNS
(It is always helpful to have your list ready before your meeting.)

Date _____ Dr. / Other _____

_____

_____

_____

_____

_____

_____

Medical
Appointment Records

❏ **DOCTOR VISITS** ❏ **OTHER SERVICES** ❏ **THERAPISTS**

(Best to use a separate page for each category.)   Year _____

Date _____Dr. / Other _____

Purpose _____

_____

Temperature_____Blood Pressure_____Pulse _____

Glucose _____Other _____Weight _____

Blood Test _____

❏ Lab   ❏ X-ray   ❏ Other Tests _____

❏ Special Referral   Dr. / Other _____

Phone (   )_____   ❏ Referral Slip   ❏ X-ray Copy

Purpose_____

_____

_____

Next Appointment: Date _____Time_____

❏ Request copy of Dr.'s report sent to Home and ❏ Other_____

Visit Summary _____

_____

_____

_____

QUESTIONS - CONCERNS
(It is always helpful to have your list ready before your meeting.)

Date _____Dr. / Other _____

_____

_____

_____

_____

_____

_____

Medical
Appointment Records

❏ **DOCTOR VISITS**   ❏ **OTHER SERVICES**   ❏ **THERAPISTS**

(Best to use a separate page for each category.)   Year _____

Date _____Dr. / Other _____

Purpose _____

_____

Temperature_____Blood Pressure_____Pulse _____

Glucose _____Other _____Weight _____

Blood Test _____

❏ Lab   ❏ X-ray   ❏ Other Tests _____

❏ Special Referral   Dr. / Other _____

Phone ( )_____   ❏ Referral Slip   ❏ X-ray Copy

Purpose_____

_____

_____

Next Appointment: Date _____Time_____

❏ Request copy of Dr.'s report sent to Home and ❏ Other_____

Visit Summary _____

_____

_____

QUESTIONS - CONCERNS
(It is always helpful to have your list ready before your meeting.)

Date _____Dr. / Other _____

_____

_____

_____

_____

_____

_____

Medical
Appointment Records

❏ **DOCTOR VISITS**   ❏ **OTHER SERVICES**   ❏ **THERAPISTS**

(Best to use a separate page for each category.)   Year _____

Date _____Dr. / Other _____

Purpose _____

_____

Temperature_____Blood Pressure_____Pulse _____

Glucose _____Other _____Weight _____

Blood Test _____

❏ Lab ❏ X-ray ❏ Other Tests _____

❏ Special Referral Dr. / Other _____

Phone (   )_____ ❏ Referral Slip ❏ X-ray Copy

Purpose_____

_____

_____

Next Appointment: Date _____Time_____

❏ Request copy of Dr.'s report sent to Home and ❏ Other_____

Visit Summary _____

_____

_____

QUESTIONS - CONCERNS
(It is always helpful to have your list ready before your meeting.)

Date _____Dr. / Other _____

_____

_____

_____

_____

_____

_____

Medical
Appointment Records

❏ **DOCTOR VISITS**   ❏ **OTHER SERVICES**   ❏ **THERAPISTS**

(Best to use a separate page for each category.)   Year _____

Date _____Dr. / Other _____

Purpose _____

_____

Temperature_____Blood Pressure_____Pulse _____

Glucose _____Other _____Weight _____

Blood Test _____

❏ Lab   ❏ X-ray   ❏ Other Tests_____

❏ Special Referral   Dr. / Other _____

Phone (   )_____   ❏ Referral Slip   ❏ X-ray Copy

Purpose_____

_____

_____

Next Appointment: Date _____Time_____

❏ Request copy of Dr.'s report sent to Home and ❏ Other_____

Visit Summary _____

_____

_____

QUESTIONS - CONCERNS
(It is always helpful to have your list ready before your meeting.)

Date _____Dr. / Other _____

_____

_____

_____

_____

_____

_____

Medical
Appointment Records

❏ **DOCTOR VISITS**　　❏ **OTHER SERVICES**　　❏ **THERAPISTS**

(Best to use a separate page for each category.)　　　　　Year _____

Date _____Dr. / Other _____

Purpose _____

_____

Temperature _____Blood Pressure _____Pulse _____

Glucose _____Other _____Weight _____

Blood Test _____

❏ Lab　❏ X-ray　❏ Other Tests _____

❏ Special Referral　Dr. / Other _____

Phone (　　)_____　❏ Referral Slip　❏ X-ray Copy

Purpose_____

_____

_____

Next Appointment:　Date _____Time_____

❏ Request copy of Dr.'s report sent to Home and ❏ Other_____

Visit Summary _____

_____

_____

QUESTIONS - CONCERNS
(It is always helpful to have your list ready before your meeting.)

Date _____Dr. / Other _____

_____

_____

_____

_____

_____

_____

Medical
Appointment Records

☐ **DOCTOR VISITS**   ☐ **OTHER SERVICES**   ☐ **THERAPISTS**

(Best to use a separate page for each category.)   Year _____

Date _____Dr. / Other _____

Purpose _____

_____

Temperature_____Blood Pressure_____Pulse _____

Glucose _____Other _____Weight _____

Blood Test _____

☐ Lab   ☐ X-ray   ☐ Other Tests _____

☐ Special Referral   Dr. / Other _____

Phone (   )_____   ☐ Referral Slip   ☐ X-ray Copy

Purpose_____

_____

_____

Next Appointment: Date _____Time_____

☐ Request copy of Dr.'s report sent to Home and ☐ Other_____

Visit Summary _____

_____

_____

QUESTIONS - CONCERNS
(It is always helpful to have your list ready before your meeting.)

Date _____Dr. / Other _____

_____

_____

_____

_____

_____

_____

Medical
Appointment Records

❑ **DOCTOR VISITS**   ❑ **OTHER SERVICES**   ❑ **THERAPISTS**

(Best to use a separate page for each category.)   Year _____

Date _____Dr. / Other _____

Purpose _____

_____

Temperature _____Blood Pressure _____Pulse _____

Glucose _____Other _____Weight _____

Blood Test _____

❑ Lab   ❑ X-ray   ❑ Other Tests _____

❑ Special Referral   Dr. / Other _____

Phone (   )_____   ❑ Referral Slip   ❑ X-ray Copy

Purpose_____

_____

_____

Next Appointment: Date _____Time_____

❑ Request copy of Dr.'s report sent to Home and ❑ Other_____

Visit Summary _____

_____

_____

QUESTIONS - CONCERNS
(It is always helpful to have your list ready before your meeting.)

Date _____Dr. / Other _____

_____

_____

_____

_____

_____

Medical
Appointment Records

❏ **DOCTOR VISITS**   ❏ **OTHER SERVICES**   ❏ **THERAPISTS**

(Best to use a separate page for each category.)   Year _____

Date _____Dr. / Other _____

Purpose _____

_____

Temperature_____Blood Pressure_____Pulse _____

Glucose _____Other _____Weight _____

Blood Test _____

❏ Lab   ❏ X-ray   ❏ Other Tests _____

❏ Special Referral   Dr. / Other _____

Phone (   )_____   ❏ Referral Slip   ❏ X-ray Copy

Purpose_____

_____

_____

Next Appointment: Date _____Time_____

❏ Request copy of Dr.'s report sent to Home and ❏ Other_____

Visit Summary _____

_____

_____

QUESTIONS - CONCERNS
(It is always helpful to have your list ready before your meeting.)

Date _____Dr. / Other _____

_____

_____

_____

_____

_____

Medical
Appointment Records

❑ **DOCTOR VISITS**   ❑ **OTHER SERVICES**   ❑ **THERAPISTS**

(Best to use a separate page for each category.)   Year _____

Date _____Dr. / Other _____

Purpose _____

_____

Temperature_____Blood Pressure_____Pulse _____

Glucose _____Other _____Weight _____

Blood Test _____

❑ Lab   ❑ X-ray   ❑ Other Tests _____

❑ Special Referral   Dr. / Other _____

Phone (   )_____   ❑ Referral Slip   ❑ X-ray Copy

Purpose_____

_____

_____

Next Appointment: Date _____Time_____

❑ Request copy of Dr.'s report sent to Home and ❑ Other_____

Visit Summary _____

_____

_____

QUESTIONS - CONCERNS
(It is always helpful to have your list ready before your meeting.)

Date _____Dr. / Other _____

_____

_____

_____

_____

_____

_____

Medical
Appointment Records

❏ **DOCTOR VISITS**   ❏ **OTHER SERVICES**   ❏ **THERAPISTS**

(Best to use a separate page for each category.)   Year _____

Date _____Dr. / Other _____

Purpose _____

_____

Temperature_____Blood Pressure_____Pulse _____

Glucose _____Other _____Weight _____

Blood Test _____

❏ Lab   ❏ X-ray   ❏ Other Tests _____

❏ Special Referral   Dr. / Other _____

Phone (   )_____   ❏ Referral Slip   ❏ X-ray Copy

Purpose_____

_____

_____

Next Appointment: Date _____Time_____

❏ Request copy of Dr.'s report sent to Home and ❏ Other_____

Visit Summary _____

_____

_____

QUESTIONS - CONCERNS
(It is always helpful to have your list ready before your meeting.)

Date _____Dr. / Other _____

_____

_____

_____

_____

_____

_____

Medical
Appointment Records

❑ **DOCTOR VISITS**   ❑ **OTHER SERVICES**   ❑ **THERAPISTS**

(Best to use a separate page for each category.)   Year _____

Date _____Dr. / Other _____

Purpose _____

_____

Temperature_____Blood Pressure_____Pulse _____

Glucose _____Other _____Weight _____

Blood Test _____

❑ Lab   ❑ X-ray   ❑ Other Tests _____

❑ Special Referral   Dr. / Other _____

Phone (   )_____   ❑ Referral Slip   ❑ X-ray Copy

Purpose_____

_____

_____

Next Appointment: Date _____Time_____

❑ Request copy of Dr.'s report sent to Home and ❑ Other_____

Visit Summary _____

_____

_____

QUESTIONS - CONCERNS
(It is always helpful to have your list ready before your meeting.)

Date _____Dr. / Other _____

_____

_____

_____

_____

_____

_____

Medical
Appointment Records

❏ **DOCTOR VISITS**   ❏ **OTHER SERVICES**   ❏ **THERAPISTS**

(Best to use a separate page for each category.)   Year _____

Date _____Dr. / Other _____

Purpose _____

_____

Temperature _____Blood Pressure_____Pulse _____

Glucose _____Other _____Weight _____

Blood Test _____

❏ Lab   ❏ X-ray   ❏ Other Tests _____

❏ Special Referral   Dr. / Other _____

Phone (   )_____   ❏ Referral Slip   ❏ X-ray Copy

Purpose_____

_____

_____

Next Appointment: Date _____Time_____

❏ Request copy of Dr.'s report sent to Home and ❏ Other_____

Visit Summary _____

_____

_____

QUESTIONS - CONCERNS
(It is always helpful to have your list ready before your meeting.)

Date _____Dr. / Other _____

_____

_____

_____

_____

_____

_____

Medical
Appointment Records

❏ **DOCTOR VISITS** ❏ **OTHER SERVICES** ❏ **THERAPISTS**

(Best to use a separate page for each category.)   Year _____

Date _____ Dr. / Other _____

Purpose _____

_____

Temperature _____ Blood Pressure _____ Pulse _____

Glucose _____ Other _____ Weight _____

Blood Test _____

❏ Lab   ❏ X-ray   ❏ Other Tests _____

❏ Special Referral   Dr. / Other _____

Phone (   ) _____   ❏ Referral Slip   ❏ X-ray Copy

Purpose _____

_____

_____

Next Appointment: Date _____ Time _____

❏ Request copy of Dr.'s report sent to Home and ❏ Other _____

Visit Summary _____

_____

_____

QUESTIONS - CONCERNS
(It is always helpful to have your list ready before your meeting.)

Date _____ Dr. / Other _____

_____

_____

_____

_____

_____

_____

Medical
Appointment Records

❏ **DOCTOR VISITS**   ❏ **OTHER SERVICES**   ❏ **THERAPISTS**

(Best to use a separate page for each category.)   Year _____

Date _____Dr. / Other _____

Purpose _____

_____

Temperature_____Blood Pressure_____Pulse _____

Glucose _____Other _____Weight _____

Blood Test _____

❏ Lab   ❏ X-ray   ❏ Other Tests _____

❏ Special Referral   Dr. / Other _____

Phone (   )_____   ❏ Referral Slip   ❏ X-ray Copy

Purpose_____

_____

_____

Next Appointment: Date _____Time_____

❏ Request copy of Dr.'s report sent to Home and ❏ Other_____

Visit Summary _____

_____

_____

QUESTIONS - CONCERNS
(It is always helpful to have your list ready before your meeting.)

Date _____Dr. / Other _____

_____

_____

_____

_____

_____

_____

_____

Medical
Appointment Records

❏ **DOCTOR VISITS**   ❏ **OTHER SERVICES**   ❏ **THERAPISTS**

(Best to use a separate page for each category.)   Year _____

Date _____ Dr. / Other _____

Purpose _____

_____

Temperature _____ Blood Pressure _____ Pulse _____

Glucose _____ Other _____ Weight _____

Blood Test _____

❏ Lab   ❏ X-ray   ❏ Other Tests _____

❏ Special Referral   Dr. / Other _____

Phone (   ) _____   ❏ Referral Slip   ❏ X-ray Copy

Purpose _____

_____

_____

Next Appointment: Date _____ Time _____

❏ Request copy of Dr.'s report sent to Home and ❏ Other _____

Visit Summary _____

_____

_____

_____

QUESTIONS - CONCERNS
(It is always helpful to have your list ready before your meeting.)

Date _____ Dr. / Other _____

_____

_____

_____

_____

_____

_____

Medical
Appointment Records

❏ **DOCTOR VISITS**   ❏ **OTHER SERVICES**   ❏ **THERAPISTS**

(Best to use a separate page for each category.)   Year _____

Date _____Dr. / Other _____

Purpose _____

_____

Temperature_____Blood Pressure_____Pulse _____

Glucose _____Other _____Weight _____

Blood Test _____

❏ Lab   ❏ X-ray   ❏ Other Tests _____

❏ Special Referral   Dr. / Other _____

Phone (   )_____   ❏ Referral Slip   ❏ X-ray Copy

Purpose_____

_____

_____

Next Appointment: Date _____Time_____

❏ Request copy of Dr.'s report sent to Home and ❏ Other_____

Visit Summary _____

_____

_____

QUESTIONS - CONCERNS
(It is always helpful to have your list ready before your meeting.)

Date _____Dr. / Other _____

_____

_____

_____

_____

_____

_____

Medical
Appointment Records

❑ **DOCTOR VISITS**   ❑ **OTHER SERVICES**   ❑ **THERAPISTS**

(Best to use a separate page for each category.)   Year _____

Date _____Dr. / Other _____

Purpose _____

_____

Temperature_____Blood Pressure_____Pulse _____

Glucose _____Other _____Weight _____

Blood Test _____

❑ Lab   ❑ X-ray   ❑ Other Tests _____

❑ Special Referral   Dr. / Other _____

Phone (   )_____   ❑ Referral Slip   ❑ X-ray Copy

Purpose_____

_____

_____

Next Appointment: Date _____Time_____

❑ Request copy of Dr.'s report sent to Home and ❑ Other_____

Visit Summary _____

_____

_____

QUESTIONS - CONCERNS
(It is always helpful to have your list ready before your meeting.)

Date _____Dr. / Other _____

_____

_____

_____

_____

_____

_____

Medical
Appointment Records

❏ **DOCTOR VISITS** ❏ **OTHER SERVICES** ❏ **THERAPISTS**

(Best to use a separate page for each category.) Year _____

Date _____Dr. / Other _____

Purpose _____

_____

Temperature_____Blood Pressure_____Pulse _____

Glucose _____Other _____Weight _____

Blood Test _____

❏ Lab ❏ X-ray ❏ Other Tests _____

❏ Special Referral   Dr. / Other _____

Phone (   )_____   ❏ Referral Slip   ❏ X-ray Copy

Purpose_____

_____

_____

Next Appointment: Date _____Time_____

❏ Request copy of Dr.'s report sent to Home and ❏ Other_____

Visit Summary _____

_____

_____

QUESTIONS - CONCERNS
(It is always helpful to have your list ready before your meeting.)

Date _____Dr. / Other _____

_____

_____

_____

_____

_____

_____

Medical
Appointment Records

❏ **DOCTOR VISITS**　　❏ **OTHER SERVICES**　　❏ **THERAPISTS**

(Best to use a separate page for each category.)　　　　　Year _____

Date _____Dr. / Other _____

Purpose _____

_____

Temperature _____Blood Pressure _____Pulse _____

Glucose _____Other _____Weight _____

Blood Test _____

❏ Lab　❏ X-ray　❏ Other Tests _____

❏ Special Referral　Dr. / Other _____

Phone (　　　)_____　❏ Referral Slip　❏ X-ray Copy

Purpose_____

_____

_____

Next Appointment:　Date _____Time_____

❏ Request copy of Dr.'s report sent to Home and ❏ Other_____

Visit Summary _____

_____

_____

QUESTIONS - CONCERNS
(It is always helpful to have your list ready before your meeting.)

Date _____Dr. / Other _____

_____

_____

_____

_____

_____

_____

Medical
Appointment Records

❏ **DOCTOR VISITS**   ❏ **OTHER SERVICES**   ❏ **THERAPISTS**

(Best to use a separate page for each category.)   Year _____

Date _____Dr. / Other _____

Purpose _____

_____

Temperature_____Blood Pressure_____Pulse _____

Glucose _____Other _____Weight _____

Blood Test _____

❏ Lab   ❏ X-ray   ❏ Other Tests _____

❏ Special Referral   Dr. / Other _____

Phone (   )_____ ❏ Referral Slip   ❏ X-ray Copy

Purpose_____

_____

_____

Next Appointment: Date _____Time_____

❏ Request copy of Dr.'s report sent to Home and ❏ Other_____

Visit Summary _____

_____

_____

_____

QUESTIONS - CONCERNS
(It is always helpful to have your list ready before your meeting.)

Date _____Dr. / Other _____

_____

_____

_____

_____

_____

_____

Medical
Appointment Records

❏ **DOCTOR VISITS**   ❏ **OTHER SERVICES**   ❏ **THERAPISTS**

(Best to use a separate page for each category.)   Year _____

Date _____Dr. / Other _____

Purpose _____

_____

Temperature_____Blood Pressure_____Pulse _____

Glucose _____Other _____Weight _____

Blood Test _____

❏ Lab   ❏ X-ray   ❏ Other Tests _____

❏ Special Referral   Dr. / Other _____

Phone (   )_____   ❏ Referral Slip   ❏ X-ray Copy

Purpose_____

_____

_____

Next Appointment: Date _____Time_____

❏ Request copy of Dr.'s report sent to Home and ❏ Other_____

Visit Summary _____

_____

_____

QUESTIONS - CONCERNS
(It is always helpful to have your list ready before your meeting.)

Date _____Dr. / Other _____

_____

_____

_____

_____

_____

_____

Medical
Appointment Records

❏ **DOCTOR VISITS**   ❏ **OTHER SERVICES**   ❏ **THERAPISTS**

(Best to use a separate page for each category.)   Year _____

Date _____ Dr. / Other _____

Purpose _____

_____

Temperature _____ Blood Pressure _____ Pulse _____

Glucose _____ Other _____ Weight _____

Blood Test _____

❏ Lab   ❏ X-ray   ❏ Other Tests _____

❏ Special Referral   Dr. / Other _____

Phone (   ) _____   ❏ Referral Slip   ❏ X-ray Copy

Purpose _____

_____

_____

Next Appointment: Date _____ Time _____

❏ Request copy of Dr.'s report sent to Home and ❏ Other_____

Visit Summary _____

_____

_____

QUESTIONS - CONCERNS
(It is always helpful to have your list ready before your meeting.)

Date _____ Dr. / Other _____

_____

_____

_____

_____

_____

_____

Medical
Appointment Records

❑ **DOCTOR VISITS**   ❑ **OTHER SERVICES**   ❑ **THERAPISTS**

(Best to use a separate page for each category.)   Year _____

Date _____Dr. / Other _____

Purpose _____

_____

Temperature _____Blood Pressure _____Pulse _____

Glucose _____Other _____Weight _____

Blood Test _____

❑ Lab   ❑ X-ray   ❑ Other Tests _____

❑ Special Referral   Dr. / Other _____

Phone (   )_____   ❑ Referral Slip   ❑ X-ray Copy

Purpose_____

_____

_____

Next Appointment: Date _____Time_____

❑ Request copy of Dr.'s report sent to Home and ❑ Other_____

Visit Summary _____

_____

_____

QUESTIONS - CONCERNS
(It is always helpful to have your list ready before your meeting.)

Date _____Dr. / Other _____

_____

_____

_____

_____

_____

_____

Medical
Appointment Records

☐ **DOCTOR VISITS**   ☐ **OTHER SERVICES**   ☐ **THERAPISTS**

(Best to use a separate page for each category.)   Year _____

Date _____ Dr. / Other _____

Purpose _____

_____

Temperature_____ Blood Pressure_____ Pulse _____

Glucose _____ Other _____ Weight _____

Blood Test _____

☐ Lab   ☐ X-ray   ☐ Other Tests _____

☐ Special Referral   Dr. / Other _____

Phone (   )_____   ☐ Referral Slip   ☐ X-ray Copy

Purpose_____

_____

_____

Next Appointment: Date _____ Time_____

☐ Request copy of Dr.'s report sent to Home and ☐ Other_____

Visit Summary _____

_____

_____

_____

QUESTIONS - CONCERNS
(It is always helpful to have your list ready before your meeting.)

Date _____ Dr. / Other _____

_____

_____

_____

_____

_____

_____

Medical
Appointment Records

❏ **DOCTOR VISITS**   ❏ **OTHER SERVICES**   ❏ **THERAPISTS**
(Best to use a separate page for each category.)   Year _____

Date _____Dr. / Other _____

Purpose _____

_____

Temperature _____Blood Pressure _____Pulse _____

Glucose _____Other _____Weight _____

Blood Test _____

❏ Lab   ❏ X-ray   ❏ Other Tests _____

❏ Special Referral   Dr. / Other _____

Phone (   ) _____   ❏ Referral Slip   ❏ X-ray Copy

Purpose _____

_____

_____

Next Appointment: Date _____Time_____

❏ Request copy of Dr.'s report sent to Home and ❏ Other_____

Visit Summary _____

_____

_____

QUESTIONS - CONCERNS
(It is always helpful to have your list ready before your meeting.)

Date _____Dr. / Other _____

_____

_____

_____

_____

_____

_____

Medical
Appointment Records

❏ **DOCTOR VISITS** ❏ **OTHER SERVICES** ❏ **THERAPISTS**

(Best to use a separate page for each category.) Year _____

Date _____ Dr. / Other _____

Purpose _____

_____

Temperature _____ Blood Pressure _____ Pulse _____

Glucose _____ Other _____ Weight _____

Blood Test _____

❏ Lab ❏ X-ray ❏ Other Tests _____

❏ Special Referral Dr. / Other _____

Phone (   ) _____ ❏ Referral Slip ❏ X-ray Copy

Purpose _____

_____

_____

Next Appointment: Date _____ Time _____

❏ Request copy of Dr.'s report sent to Home and ❏ Other _____

Visit Summary _____

_____

_____

QUESTIONS - CONCERNS
(It is always helpful to have your list ready before your meeting.)

Date _____ Dr. / Other _____

_____

_____

_____

_____

_____

_____

Medical
Appointment Records

❏ **DOCTOR VISITS**   ❏ **OTHER SERVICES**   ❏ **THERAPISTS**

(Best to use a separate page for each category.)   Year _____

Date _____ Dr. / Other _____

Purpose _____

_____

Temperature _____ Blood Pressure _____ Pulse _____

Glucose _____ Other _____ Weight _____

Blood Test _____

❏ Lab   ❏ X-ray   ❏ Other Tests _____

❏ Special Referral   Dr. / Other _____

Phone (   ) _____   ❏ Referral Slip   ❏ X-ray Copy

Purpose _____

_____

_____

Next Appointment: Date _____ Time _____

❏ Request copy of Dr.'s report sent to Home and ❏ Other_____

Visit Summary _____

_____

_____

_____

QUESTIONS - CONCERNS
(It is always helpful to have your list ready before your meeting.)

Date _____ Dr. / Other _____

_____

_____

_____

_____

_____

_____

Medical
Appointment Records

❏ **DOCTOR VISITS** ❏ **OTHER SERVICES** ❏ **THERAPISTS**

(Best to use a separate page for each category.) Year _____

Date _____Dr. / Other _____

Purpose _____

_____

Temperature_____Blood Pressure_____Pulse _____

Glucose _____Other _____Weight _____

Blood Test _____

❏ Lab ❏ X-ray ❏ Other Tests _____

❏ Special Referral Dr. / Other _____

Phone ( )_____ ❏ Referral Slip ❏ X-ray Copy

Purpose_____

_____

_____

Next Appointment: Date _____Time_____

❏ Request copy of Dr.'s report sent to Home and ❏ Other_____

Visit Summary _____

_____

_____

QUESTIONS - CONCERNS
(It is always helpful to have your list ready before your meeting.)

Date _____Dr. / Other _____

_____

_____

_____

_____

_____

_____

Medical
Appointment Records

❏ **DOCTOR VISITS**   ❏ **OTHER SERVICES**   ❏ **THERAPISTS**

(Best to use a separate page for each category.)   Year _____

Date _____ Dr. / Other _____

Purpose _____

_____

Temperature _____ Blood Pressure _____ Pulse _____

Glucose _____ Other _____ Weight _____

Blood Test _____

❏ Lab   ❏ X-ray   ❏ Other Tests _____

❏ Special Referral   Dr. / Other _____

Phone (   ) _____   ❏ Referral Slip   ❏ X-ray Copy

Purpose_____

_____

_____

Next Appointment: Date _____ Time _____

❏ Request copy of Dr.'s report sent to Home and ❏ Other_____

Visit Summary _____

_____

_____

_____

QUESTIONS - CONCERNS
(It is always helpful to have your list ready before your meeting.)

Date _____ Dr. / Other _____

_____

_____

_____

_____

_____

_____

Medical
Appointment Records

☐ **DOCTOR VISITS**   ☐ **OTHER SERVICES**   ☐ **THERAPISTS**

(Best to use a separate page for each category.)   Year _____

Date _____ Dr. / Other _____

Purpose _____

_____

Temperature _____ Blood Pressure _____ Pulse _____

Glucose _____ Other _____ Weight _____

Blood Test _____

☐ Lab   ☐ X-ray   ☐ Other Tests _____

☐ Special Referral   Dr. / Other _____

Phone (____) _____   ☐ Referral Slip   ☐ X-ray Copy

Purpose _____

_____

_____

Next Appointment: Date _____ Time_____

☐ Request copy of Dr.'s report sent to Home and ☐ Other_____

Visit Summary _____

_____

_____

_____

QUESTIONS - CONCERNS
(It is always helpful to have your list ready before your meeting.)

Date _____ Dr. / Other _____

_____

_____

_____

_____

_____

_____

Medical
Appointment Records

❏ **DOCTOR VISITS**   ❏ **OTHER SERVICES**   ❏ **THERAPISTS**

(Best to use a separate page for each category.)   Year _____

Date _____Dr. / Other _____

Purpose _____

_____

Temperature_____Blood Pressure_____Pulse _____

Glucose _____Other _____Weight _____

Blood Test _____

❏ Lab   ❏ X-ray   ❏ Other Tests _____

❏ Special Referral   Dr. / Other _____

Phone (   )_____   ❏ Referral Slip   ❏ X-ray Copy

Purpose_____

_____

_____

Next Appointment: Date _____Time_____

❏ Request copy of Dr.'s report sent to Home and ❏ Other_____

Visit Summary _____

_____

_____

QUESTIONS - CONCERNS
(It is always helpful to have your list ready before your meeting.)

Date _____Dr. / Other _____

_____

_____

_____

_____

_____

_____

Medical
Appointment Records

❏ **DOCTOR VISITS**   ❏ **OTHER SERVICES**   ❏ **THERAPISTS**

(Best to use a separate page for each category.)   Year _____

Date _____Dr. / Other _____

Purpose _____

_____

Temperature_____Blood Pressure_____Pulse _____

Glucose _____Other _____Weight _____

Blood Test _____

❏ Lab   ❏ X-ray   ❏ Other Tests _____

❏ Special Referral   Dr. / Other _____

Phone (   )_____   ❏ Referral Slip   ❏ X-ray Copy

Purpose_____

_____

_____

Next Appointment: Date _____Time_____

❏ Request copy of Dr.'s report sent to Home and ❏ Other_____

Visit Summary _____

_____

_____

QUESTIONS - CONCERNS
(It is always helpful to have your list ready before your meeting.)

Date _____Dr. / Other _____

_____

_____

_____

_____

_____

_____

Medical
Appointment Records

❏ **DOCTOR VISITS**   ❏ **OTHER SERVICES**   ❏ **THERAPISTS**

(Best to use a separate page for each category.)   Year _____

Date _____ Dr. / Other _____

Purpose _____

_____

Temperature _____ Blood Pressure _____ Pulse _____

Glucose _____ Other _____ Weight _____

Blood Test _____

❏ Lab   ❏ X-ray   ❏ Other Tests _____

❏ Special Referral   Dr. / Other _____

Phone (   ) _____ ❏ Referral Slip ❏ X-ray Copy

Purpose _____

_____

_____

Next Appointment: Date _____ Time _____

❏ Request copy of Dr.'s report sent to Home and ❏ Other_____

Visit Summary _____

_____

_____

_____

QUESTIONS - CONCERNS
(It is always helpful to have your list ready before your meeting.)

Date _____ Dr. / Other _____

_____

_____

_____

_____

_____

_____

Medical
Appointment Records

❑ **DOCTOR VISITS**   ❑ **OTHER SERVICES**   ❑ **THERAPISTS**
(Best to use a separate page for each category.)   Year _____

Date _____Dr. / Other _____

Purpose _____

_____

Temperature_____Blood Pressure_____Pulse _____

Glucose _____Other _____Weight _____

Blood Test _____

❑ Lab   ❑ X-ray   ❑ Other Tests _____

❑ Special Referral   Dr. / Other _____

Phone (   )_____   ❑ Referral Slip   ❑ X-ray Copy

Purpose_____

_____

_____

Next Appointment: Date _____Time_____

❑ Request copy of Dr.'s report sent to Home and ❑ Other_____

Visit Summary _____

_____

_____

_____

QUESTIONS - CONCERNS
(It is always helpful to have your list ready before your meeting.)

Date _____Dr. / Other _____

_____

_____

_____

_____

_____

_____

147

Medical
Appointment Records

❑ **DOCTOR VISITS**   ❑ **OTHER SERVICES**   ❑ **THERAPISTS**

(Best to use a separate page for each category.)   Year _____

Date _____Dr. / Other _____

Purpose _____

_____

Temperature_____Blood Pressure_____Pulse _____

Glucose _____Other _____Weight _____

Blood Test _____

❑ Lab   ❑ X-ray   ❑ Other Tests _____

❑ Special Referral   Dr. / Other _____

Phone (   )_____   ❑ Referral Slip   ❑ X-ray Copy

Purpose_____

_____

_____

Next Appointment: Date _____Time_____

❑ Request copy of Dr.'s report sent to Home and ❑ Other_____

Visit Summary _____

_____

_____

_____

QUESTIONS - CONCERNS
(It is always helpful to have your list ready before your meeting.)

Date _____Dr. / Other _____

_____

_____

_____

_____

_____

_____

Dental
Appointment Records

Dental Appointments: This is especially helpful for your dentist when you are referred to a specialist or another dentist.

Notes

Dental Appointments

Dental Appointment Records

❏ **DOCTOR VISITS**   ❏ **OTHER SERVICES**

(Best to use a separate page for each category.)

Year _____

Date _____Dr. / Other _____

Purpose _____

_____

Treatment Plan _____ ❏ Pending   ❏ Type: _____

Treatment Summary _____

❏ Lab   ❏ X-ray   ❏ Dental Impressions Type _____

Next Appointment: Date _____   Time _____

❏ Request copy of Dr.'s report sent to Home and ❏ Other _____

❏ Special Referral   Dr. / Other_____

Phone (   )_____ ❏ Referral Slip   ❏ X-ray Copy

Purpose _____

_____

Visit Summary _____

_____

_____

QUESTIONS - CONCERNS

(It is always helpful to have your list ready before your meeting.)

Date _____Dr. / Other _____

_____

_____

_____

_____

_____

_____

Dental Appointment Records

❏ DOCTOR VISITS   ❏ OTHER SERVICES

(Best to use a separate page for each category.)

Year _____

Date _____ Dr. / Other _____

Purpose _____

_____

Treatment Plan _____ ❏ Pending   ❏ Type: _____

   Treatment Summary _____

❏ Lab   ❏ X-ray   ❏ Dental Impressions Type _____

Next Appointment: Date _____ Time _____

❏ Request copy of Dr.'s report sent to Home and ❏ Other _____

❏ Special Referral   Dr. / Other_____

Phone (   )_____ ❏ Referral Slip   ❏ X-ray Copy

Purpose _____

_____

Visit Summary _____

_____

_____

QUESTIONS - CONCERNS

(It is always helpful to have your list ready before your meeting.)

Date _____ Dr. / Other _____

_____

_____

_____

_____

_____

_____

Dental Appointments

Dental Appointment Records

❑ **DOCTOR VISITS**   ❑ **OTHER SERVICES**
(Best to use a separate page for each category.)

Year _____

Date _____Dr. / Other _____

Purpose _____

_____

Treatment Plan _____❑ Pending   ❑ Type: _____

      Treatment Summary _____

❑ Lab   ❑ X-ray   ❑ Dental Impressions Type _____

Next Appointment: Date _____ Time _____

❑ Request copy of Dr.'s report sent to Home and ❑ Other _____

❑ Special Referral   Dr. / Other_____

Phone (   )_____ ❑ Referral Slip   ❑ X-ray Copy

Purpose _____

_____

Visit Summary _____

_____

_____

QUESTIONS - CONCERNS

(It is always helpful to have your list ready before your meeting.)

Date _____Dr. / Other _____

_____

_____

_____

_____

_____

_____

Dental Appointments

Dental Appointment Records

Dental Appointments

❏ **DOCTOR VISITS**   ❏ **OTHER SERVICES**

(Best to use a separate page for each category.)

Year _____

Date _____ Dr. / Other _____

Purpose _____

_____

Treatment Plan _____❏ Pending   ❏ Type: _____

   Treatment Summary _____

❏ Lab   ❏ X-ray   ❏ Dental Impressions Type _____

Next Appointment: Date _____ Time _____

❏ Request copy of Dr.'s report sent to Home and ❏ Other _____

❏ Special Referral   Dr. / Other_____

Phone (   )_____ ❏ Referral Slip   ❏ X-ray Copy

Purpose _____

_____

Visit Summary _____

_____

_____

QUESTIONS - CONCERNS

(It is always helpful to have your list ready before your meeting.)

Date _____ Dr. / Other _____

_____

_____

_____

_____

_____

_____

Dental Appointment Records

❏ **DOCTOR VISITS**   ❏ **OTHER SERVICES**
(Best to use a separate page for each category.)

Year _____

Date _____ Dr. / Other _____

Purpose _____

_____

Treatment Plan _____ ❏ Pending   ❏ Type: _____

    Treatment Summary _____

❏ Lab   ❏ X-ray   ❏ Dental Impressions Type _____

Next Appointment: Date _____ Time _____

❏ Request copy of Dr.'s report sent to Home and ❏ Other _____

❏ Special Referral   Dr. / Other_____

Phone (   )_____ ❏ Referral Slip   ❏ X-ray Copy

Purpose _____

_____

Visit Summary _____

_____

_____

_____

QUESTIONS - CONCERNS

(It is always helpful to have your list ready before your meeting.)

Date _____ Dr. / Other _____

_____

_____

_____

_____

_____

_____

© 2008 Life Cycles Publishing, Inc. All Rights Reserved.

Dental Appointments

Dental Appointment Records

❏ DOCTOR VISITS   ❏ OTHER SERVICES

(Best to use a separate page for each category.)

Year _____

Date _____ Dr. / Other _____

Purpose _____

_____

Treatment Plan _____ ❏ Pending   ❏ Type: _____

    Treatment Summary _____

❏ Lab   ❏ X-ray   ❏ Dental Impressions Type _____

Next Appointment: Date _____   Time _____

❏ Request copy of Dr.'s report sent to Home and ❏ Other _____

❏ Special Referral   Dr. / Other_____

Phone (   )_____ ❏ Referral Slip   ❏ X-ray Copy

Purpose _____

_____

Visit Summary _____

_____

_____

QUESTIONS - CONCERNS

(It is always helpful to have your list ready before your meeting.)

Date _____ Dr. / Other _____

_____

_____

_____

_____

_____

Dental Appointments

Dental Appointment Records

❏ **DOCTOR VISITS**   ❏ **OTHER SERVICES**
(Best to use a separate page for each category.)

Year _____

Date _____Dr. / Other _____

Purpose _____

_____

Treatment Plan _____❏ Pending   ❏ Type: _____

    Treatment Summary _____

❏ Lab   ❏ X-ray   ❏ Dental Impressions Type _____

Next Appointment: Date _____ Time _____

❏ Request copy of Dr.'s report sent to Home and ❏ Other _____

❏ Special Referral   Dr. / Other_____

Phone (   )_____ ❏ Referral Slip   ❏ X-ray Copy

Purpose _____

_____

Visit Summary _____

_____

_____

QUESTIONS - CONCERNS

(It is always helpful to have your list ready before your meeting.)

Date _____Dr. / Other _____

_____

_____

_____

_____

_____

_____

Dental Appointments

Dental Appointment Records

❏ **DOCTOR VISITS**   ❏ **OTHER SERVICES**

(Best to use a separate page for each category.)

Year _____

Date _____Dr. / Other _____

Purpose _____

_____

Treatment Plan _____❏ Pending   ❏ Type: _____

  Treatment Summary _____

❏ Lab   ❏ X-ray   ❏ Dental Impressions Type _____

Next Appointment: Date _____ Time _____

❏ Request copy of Dr.'s report sent to Home and ❏ Other _____

❏ Special Referral   Dr. / Other_____

Phone (   )_____ ❏ Referral Slip   ❏ X-ray Copy

Purpose _____

_____

Visit Summary _____

_____

_____

QUESTIONS - CONCERNS

(It is always helpful to have your list ready before your meeting.)

Date _____Dr. / Other _____

_____

_____

_____

_____

_____

Dental Appointments

Dental Appointment Records

❏ **DOCTOR VISITS**   ❏ **OTHER SERVICES**

(Best to use a separate page for each category.)

Year _____

Date _____ Dr. / Other _____

Purpose _____

_____

Treatment Plan _____❏ Pending   ❏ Type: _____

   Treatment Summary _____

❏ Lab   ❏ X-ray   ❏ Dental Impressions Type _____

Next Appointment: Date _____ Time _____

❏ Request copy of Dr.'s report sent to Home and ❏ Other _____

❏ Special Referral   Dr. / Other_____

Phone (   )_____ ❏ Referral Slip   ❏ X-ray Copy

Purpose _____

_____

Visit Summary _____

_____

_____

QUESTIONS - CONCERNS

(It is always helpful to have your list ready before your meeting.)

Date _____ Dr. / Other _____

_____

_____

_____

_____

_____

_____

Dental Appointment Records

☐ **DOCTOR VISITS**   ☐ **OTHER SERVICES**

(Best to use a separate page for each category.)

Year _____

Date _____Dr. / Other _____

Purpose _____

_____

Treatment Plan _____☐ Pending   ☐ Type: _____

  Treatment Summary _____

☐ Lab   ☐ X-ray   ☐ Dental Impressions Type _____

Next Appointment: Date _____ Time _____

☐ Request copy of Dr.'s report sent to Home and ☐ Other _____

☐ Special Referral   Dr. / Other_____

Phone (   )_____ ☐ Referral Slip   ☐ X-ray Copy

Purpose _____

_____

Visit Summary _____

_____

_____

QUESTIONS - CONCERNS

(It is always helpful to have your list ready before your meeting.)

Date _____Dr. / Other _____

_____

_____

_____

_____

_____

_____

Dental Appointments

Dental Appointment Records

❏ **DOCTOR VISITS** ❏ **OTHER SERVICES**

(Best to use a separate page for each category.)

Year _____

Date _____ Dr. / Other _____

Purpose _____

_____

Treatment Plan _____❏ Pending ❏ Type: _____

   Treatment Summary _____

❏ Lab ❏ X-ray ❏ Dental Impressions Type _____

Next Appointment: Date _____ Time _____

❏ Request copy of Dr.'s report sent to Home and ❏ Other _____

❏ Special Referral Dr. / Other_____

Phone ( ) _____ ❏ Referral Slip ❏ X-ray Copy

Purpose _____

_____

Visit Summary _____

_____

_____

QUESTIONS - CONCERNS

(It is always helpful to have your list ready before your meeting.)

Date _____ Dr. / Other _____

_____

_____

_____

_____

_____

_____

Dental Appointments

Dental Appointment Records

❏ **DOCTOR VISITS**   ❏ **OTHER SERVICES**

(Best to use a separate page for each category.)

Year _____

Date _____Dr. / Other _____

Purpose _____

_____

Treatment Plan _____❏ Pending   ❏ Type: _____

   Treatment Summary _____

❏ Lab   ❏ X-ray   ❏ Dental Impressions Type _____

Next Appointment: Date _____ Time _____

❏ Request copy of Dr.'s report sent to Home and ❏ Other _____

❏ Special Referral   Dr. / Other_____

Phone (   )_____ ❏ Referral Slip   ❏ X-ray Copy

Purpose _____

_____

Visit Summary _____

_____

_____

QUESTIONS - CONCERNS

(It is always helpful to have your list ready before your meeting.)

Date _____Dr. / Other _____

_____

_____

_____

_____

_____

_____

Dental Appointments

Dental Appointment Records

❏ **DOCTOR VISITS**   ❏ **OTHER SERVICES**

(Best to use a separate page for each category.)

Year _____

Date _____Dr. / Other _____

Purpose _____

_____

Treatment Plan _____❏ Pending ❏ Type: _____

    Treatment Summary _____

❏ Lab ❏ X-ray ❏ Dental Impressions Type _____

Next Appointment: Date _____ Time _____

❏ Request copy of Dr.'s report sent to Home and ❏ Other _____

❏ Special Referral Dr. / Other_____

Phone (   ) _____ ❏ Referral Slip   ❏ X-ray Copy

Purpose _____

_____

Visit Summary _____

_____

_____

QUESTIONS - CONCERNS

(It is always helpful to have your list ready before your meeting.)

Date _____Dr. / Other _____

_____

_____

_____

_____

_____

_____

Dental Appointment Records

❏ DOCTOR VISITS   ❏ OTHER SERVICES

(Best to use a separate page for each category.)

Year _____

Date _____Dr. / Other _____

Purpose _____

_____

Treatment Plan _____❏ Pending   ❏ Type: _____

   Treatment Summary _____

❏ Lab   ❏ X-ray   ❏ Dental Impressions Type _____

Next Appointment: Date _____   Time _____

❏ Request copy of Dr.'s report sent to Home and ❏ Other _____

❏ Special Referral   Dr. / Other_____

Phone (   )_____ ❏ Referral Slip   ❏ X-ray Copy

Purpose _____

_____

Visit Summary _____

_____

_____

QUESTIONS - CONCERNS

(It is always helpful to have your list ready before your meeting.)

Date _____Dr. / Other _____

_____

_____

_____

_____

_____

_____

Dental Appointments

Dental Appointment Records

❏ **DOCTOR VISITS**　　❏ **OTHER SERVICES**

(Best to use a separate page for each category.)

Year _____

Date _____Dr. / Other _____

Purpose _____

_____

Treatment Plan _____❏ Pending　❏ Type: _____

　　Treatment Summary _____

❏ Lab　❏ X-ray　❏ Dental Impressions Type _____

Next Appointment:　Date _____ Time _____

❏ Request copy of Dr.'s report sent to Home and ❏ Other _____

❏ Special Referral　Dr. / Other_____

Phone (　　　)_____ ❏ Referral Slip　❏ X-ray Copy

Purpose _____

_____

Visit Summary _____

_____

_____

QUESTIONS - CONCERNS

(It is always helpful to have your list ready before your meeting.)

Date _____Dr. / Other _____

_____

_____

_____

_____

_____

_____

Dental Appointments

Dental Appointment Records

❏ **DOCTOR VISITS**   ❏ **OTHER SERVICES**

(Best to use a separate page for each category.)

Year _____

Date _____ Dr. / Other _____

Purpose _____

_____

Treatment Plan _____ ❏ Pending   ❏ Type: _____

   Treatment Summary _____

❏ Lab   ❏ X-ray   ❏ Dental Impressions Type _____

Next Appointment: Date _____ Time _____

❏ Request copy of Dr.'s report sent to Home and ❏ Other _____

❏ Special Referral   Dr. / Other_____

Phone (   )_____ ❏ Referral Slip   ❏ X-ray Copy

Purpose _____

_____

Visit Summary _____

_____

_____

QUESTIONS - CONCERNS

(It is always helpful to have your list ready before your meeting.)

Date _____ Dr. / Other _____

_____

_____

_____

_____

_____

_____

Dental Appointments *(sidebar tab)*

Dental Appointment Records

☐ **DOCTOR VISITS**   ☐ **OTHER SERVICES**

(Best to use a separate page for each category.)

Year _____

Date _____Dr. / Other _____

Purpose _____

_____

Treatment Plan _____☐ Pending   ☐ Type: _____

  Treatment Summary _____

☐ Lab   ☐ X-ray   ☐ Dental Impressions Type _____

Next Appointment: Date _____ Time _____

☐ Request copy of Dr.'s report sent to Home and ☐ Other _____

☐ Special Referral   Dr. / Other_____

Phone (   )_____ ☐ Referral Slip   ☐ X-ray Copy

Purpose _____

_____

Visit Summary _____

_____

_____

QUESTIONS - CONCERNS

(It is always helpful to have your list ready before your meeting.)

Date _____Dr. / Other _____

_____

_____

_____

_____

_____

_____

Dental Appointments

Dental Appointment Records

❏ **DOCTOR VISITS**   ❏ **OTHER SERVICES**

(Best to use a separate page for each category.)

Year _____

Date _____Dr. / Other _____

Purpose _____

_____

Treatment Plan _____❏ Pending   ❏ Type: _____

    Treatment Summary _____

❏ Lab   ❏ X-ray   ❏ Dental Impressions Type _____

Next Appointment: Date _____ Time _____

❏ Request copy of Dr.'s report sent to Home and ❏ Other _____

❏ Special Referral   Dr. / Other_____

Phone (   )_____ ❏ Referral Slip   ❏ X-ray Copy

Purpose _____

_____

Visit Summary _____

_____

_____

QUESTIONS - CONCERNS

(It is always helpful to have your list ready before your meeting.)

Date _____Dr. / Other _____

_____

_____

_____

_____

_____

_____

Dental Appointments

Dental Appointment Records

❑ **DOCTOR VISITS**   ❑ **OTHER SERVICES**

(Best to use a separate page for each category.)

Year _____

Date _____Dr. / Other _____

Purpose _____

_____

Treatment Plan _____❑ Pending   ❑ Type: _____

  Treatment Summary _____

❑ Lab   ❑ X-ray   ❑ Dental Impressions Type _____

Next Appointment: Date _____ Time _____

❑ Request copy of Dr.'s report sent to Home and ❑ Other _____

❑ Special Referral   Dr. / Other_____

Phone (   )_____ ❑ Referral Slip   ❑ X-ray Copy

Purpose _____

_____

Visit Summary _____

_____

_____

QUESTIONS - CONCERNS

(It is always helpful to have your list ready before your meeting.)

Date _____Dr. / Other _____

_____

_____

_____

_____

_____

_____

Dental Appointments

169

Dental Appointment Records

❏ DOCTOR VISITS   ❏ OTHER SERVICES

(Best to use a separate page for each category.)

Year _____

Date _____Dr. / Other _____

Purpose _____

_____

Treatment Plan _____❏ Pending   ❏ Type: _____

    Treatment Summary _____

❏ Lab   ❏ X-ray   ❏ Dental Impressions Type _____

Next Appointment: Date _____ Time _____

❏ Request copy of Dr.'s report sent to Home and ❏ Other _____

❏ Special Referral   Dr. / Other_____

Phone (   )_____ ❏ Referral Slip   ❏ X-ray Copy

Purpose _____

_____

Visit Summary _____

_____

_____

QUESTIONS - CONCERNS

(It is always helpful to have your list ready before your meeting.)

Date _____Dr. / Other _____

_____

_____

_____

_____

_____

_____

Dental Appointments (sidebar)

Dental Appointment Records

☐ **DOCTOR VISITS**   ☐ **OTHER SERVICES**

(Best to use a separate page for each category.)

Year _____

Date _____ Dr. / Other _____

Purpose _____

_____

Treatment Plan _____☐ Pending   ☐ Type: _____

    Treatment Summary _____

☐ Lab   ☐ X-ray   ☐ Dental Impressions Type _____

Next Appointment: Date _____ Time _____

☐ Request copy of Dr.'s report sent to Home and ☐ Other _____

☐ Special Referral   Dr. / Other_____

Phone (   )_____ ☐ Referral Slip   ☐ X-ray Copy

Purpose _____

_____

Visit Summary _____

_____

_____

QUESTIONS - CONCERNS

(It is always helpful to have your list ready before your meeting.)

Date _____ Dr. / Other _____

_____

_____

_____

_____

_____

_____

Dental Appointment Records

❏ **DOCTOR VISITS**   ❏ **OTHER SERVICES**

(Best to use a separate page for each category.)

Year _____

Date _____ Dr. / Other _____

Purpose _____

_____

Treatment Plan _____❏ Pending   ❏ Type: _____

   Treatment Summary _____

❏ Lab   ❏ X-ray   ❏ Dental Impressions Type _____

Next Appointment: Date _____   Time _____

❏ Request copy of Dr.'s report sent to Home and ❏ Other _____

❏ Special Referral   Dr. / Other_____

Phone (   )_____ ❏ Referral Slip   ❏ X-ray Copy

Purpose _____

_____

Visit Summary _____

_____

_____

QUESTIONS - CONCERNS

(It is always helpful to have your list ready before your meeting.)

Date _____ Dr. / Other _____

_____

_____

_____

_____

_____

_____

Dental Appointments *(side tab)*

Dental Appointment Records

❏ **DOCTOR VISITS** ❏ **OTHER SERVICES**

(Best to use a separate page for each category.)

Year _____

Date _____Dr. / Other _____

Purpose _____

_____

Treatment Plan _____❏ Pending ❏ Type: _____

　　Treatment Summary _____

❏ Lab ❏ X-ray ❏ Dental Impressions Type _____

Next Appointment: Date _____ Time _____

❏ Request copy of Dr.'s report sent to Home and ❏ Other _____

❏ Special Referral Dr. / Other_____

Phone (   )_____ ❏ Referral Slip   ❏ X-ray Copy

Purpose _____

_____

Visit Summary _____

_____

_____

QUESTIONS - CONCERNS

(It is always helpful to have your list ready before your meeting.)

Date _____Dr. / Other _____

_____

_____

_____

_____

_____

_____

Dental Appointments

Dental Appointment Records

❏ **DOCTOR VISITS**   ❏ **OTHER SERVICES**

(Best to use a separate page for each category.)

Year _____

Date _____Dr. / Other _____

Purpose _____

_____

Treatment Plan _____❏ Pending ❏ Type: _____

   Treatment Summary _____

❏ Lab ❏ X-ray ❏ Dental Impressions Type _____

Next Appointment: Date _____ Time _____

❏ Request copy of Dr.'s report sent to Home and ❏ Other _____

❏ Special Referral Dr. / Other_____

Phone (_____)_____ ❏ Referral Slip   ❏ X-ray Copy

Purpose _____

_____

Visit Summary _____

_____

_____

QUESTIONS - CONCERNS

(It is always helpful to have your list ready before your meeting.)

Date _____Dr. / Other _____

_____

_____

_____

_____

_____

_____

Dental Appointments

Dental Appointment Records

☐ **DOCTOR VISITS**   ☐ **OTHER SERVICES**

(Best to use a separate page for each category.)

Year _____

Date _____Dr. / Other _____

Purpose _____

_____

Treatment Plan _____☐ Pending   ☐ Type: _____

   Treatment Summary _____

☐ Lab   ☐ X-ray   ☐ Dental Impressions Type _____

Next Appointment: Date _____   Time _____

☐ Request copy of Dr.'s report sent to Home and ☐ Other _____

☐ Special Referral   Dr. / Other_____

Phone (   )_____ ☐ Referral Slip   ☐ X-ray Copy

Purpose _____

_____

Visit Summary _____

_____

_____

QUESTIONS - CONCERNS

(It is always helpful to have your list ready before your meeting.)

Date _____Dr. / Other _____

_____

_____

_____

_____

_____

_____

Dental Appointments

Dental Appointment Records

❏ DOCTOR VISITS   ❏ OTHER SERVICES

(Best to use a separate page for each category.)

Year _____

Date _____Dr. / Other _____

Purpose _____

_____

Treatment Plan _____❏ Pending   ❏ Type: _____

   Treatment Summary _____

❏ Lab   ❏ X-ray   ❏ Dental Impressions Type _____

Next Appointment: Date _____ Time _____

❏ Request copy of Dr.'s report sent to Home and ❏ Other _____

❏ Special Referral   Dr. / Other_____

Phone (   )_____ ❏ Referral Slip   ❏ X-ray Copy

Purpose _____

_____

Visit Summary _____

_____

_____

QUESTIONS - CONCERNS

(It is always helpful to have your list ready before your meeting.)

Date _____Dr. / Other _____

_____

_____

_____

_____

_____

_____

Dental Appointments

Dental Appointment Records

☐ **DOCTOR VISITS**   ☐ **OTHER SERVICES**

(Best to use a separate page for each category.)

Year _____

Date _____Dr. / Other _____

Purpose _____

_____

Treatment Plan _____☐ Pending   ☐ Type: _____

   Treatment Summary _____

☐ Lab   ☐ X-ray   ☐ Dental Impressions Type _____

Next Appointment: Date _____ Time _____

☐ Request copy of Dr.'s report sent to Home and ☐ Other _____

☐ Special Referral   Dr. / Other_____

Phone (   )_____ ☐ Referral Slip   ☐ X-ray Copy

Purpose _____

_____

Visit Summary _____

_____

_____

QUESTIONS - CONCERNS

(It is always helpful to have your list ready before your meeting.)

Date _____Dr. / Other _____

_____

_____

_____

_____

_____

_____

Dental Appointments

Dental Appointment Records

❏ DOCTOR VISITS   ❏ OTHER SERVICES

(Best to use a separate page for each category.)

Year _____

Date _____Dr. / Other _____

Purpose _____

_____

Treatment Plan _____❏ Pending   ❏ Type: _____

    Treatment Summary _____

❏ Lab   ❏ X-ray   ❏ Dental Impressions Type _____

Next Appointment: Date _____ Time _____

❏ Request copy of Dr.'s report sent to Home and ❏ Other _____

❏ Special Referral   Dr. / Other_____

Phone (   )_____ ❏ Referral Slip   ❏ X-ray Copy

Purpose _____

_____

Visit Summary _____

_____

_____

QUESTIONS - CONCERNS

(It is always helpful to have your list ready before your meeting.)

Date _____Dr. / Other _____

_____

_____

_____

_____

_____

_____

Dental Appointments

Dental Appointment Records

❏ **DOCTOR VISITS**   ❏ **OTHER SERVICES**

(Best to use a separate page for each category.)

Year _____

Date _____ Dr. / Other _____

Purpose _____

_____

Treatment Plan _____❏ Pending   ❏ Type: _____

   Treatment Summary _____

❏ Lab   ❏ X-ray   ❏ Dental Impressions Type _____

Next Appointment: Date _____ Time _____

❏ Request copy of Dr.'s report sent to Home and ❏ Other _____

❏ Special Referral   Dr. / Other_____

Phone (   )_____ ❏ Referral Slip   ❏ X-ray Copy

Purpose _____

_____

Visit Summary _____

_____

_____

QUESTIONS - CONCERNS

(It is always helpful to have your list ready before your meeting.)

Date _____ Dr. / Other _____

_____

_____

_____

_____

_____

_____

Dental Appointments

Dental Appointment Records

❑ DOCTOR VISITS   ❑ OTHER SERVICES

(Best to use a separate page for each category.)

Year _____

Date _____Dr. / Other _____

Purpose _____

_____

Treatment Plan _____❑ Pending   ❑ Type: _____

   Treatment Summary _____

❑ Lab   ❑ X-ray   ❑ Dental Impressions Type _____

Next Appointment: Date _____ Time _____

❑ Request copy of Dr.'s report sent to Home and ❑ Other _____

❑ Special Referral   Dr. / Other_____

Phone (   )_____ ❑ Referral Slip   ❑ X-ray Copy

Purpose _____

_____

Visit Summary _____

_____

_____

QUESTIONS - CONCERNS

(It is always helpful to have your list ready before your meeting.)

Date _____Dr. / Other _____

_____

_____

_____

_____

_____

_____

Dental Appointments

Laboratory Work * X-Ray Log
Laboratory Work * X-Ray Records

Laboratory Work * X-ray: State the type of test, the reason for it and the results. Depending on the test, request a copy of the report and/or x-ray for your file. This is helpful especially for future reference and to assist any professional when evaluating a medical treatment or condition. If the service provider will not release the report to you, you will need to request that it to be sent to your physician. Then you can request a copy from your physician.

Notes

Laboratory Work * X-Ray

Laboratory Work ∗ X-Ray Log

Place a (✓) in the appropriate category.

DATE	TYPE	X-RAY	BLOOD TEST	PROCEDURE	OTHER	COMMENTS

Laboratory Work ∗ X-Ray

Laboratory Work * X-Ray Log

Place a (✓) in the appropriate category.

DATE	TYPE	X-RAY	BLOOD TEST	PROCEDURE	OTHER	COMMENTS

Laboratory Work * X-Ray

Laboratory Work * X-Ray Log

Place a (✓) in the appropriate category.

DATE	TYPE	X-RAY	BLOOD TEST	PROCEDURE	OTHER	COMMENTS

Laboratory Work * X-Ray

Laboratory Work * X-Ray Log

Place a (✓) in the appropriate category.

DATE	TYPE	X-RAY	BLOOD TEST	PROCEDURE	OTHER	COMMENTS

Laboratory Work * X-Ray

Laboratory Work * X-Ray Log

❏ LABORATORY WORK ❏ X-RAY

(Best to use a separate page for each category.)

Date _____ Phone (___) _____

Facility _____

Address _____

City _____ State _____ Zip _____

Requested by _____ Dr. _____

Purpose _____

_____

Request copy of: ❏ Report   ❏ X-rays   ❏ Lab Results   ❏ Other _____

Prepare for test: ❏ No   ❏ Yes _____

Note _____

_____

_____

Date _____ Phone (___) _____

Facility _____

Address _____

City _____ State _____ Zip _____

Requested by _____ Dr. _____

Purpose _____

_____

Request copy of: ❏ Report   ❏ X-rays   ❏ Lab Results   ❏ Other _____

Prepare for test: ❏ No   ❏ Yes _____

Note _____

_____

_____

Laboratory Work * X-Ray Log

❏ **LABORATORY WORK**　　❏ **X-RAY**
(Best to use a separate page for each category.)

Date _____Phone (   ) _____

Facility_____

Address _____

City _____ State _____ Zip_____

Requested by _____Dr. _____

Purpose _____

_____

Request copy of: ❏ Report　❏ X-rays　❏ Lab Results　❏ Other _____

Prepare for test: ❏ No　　❏ Yes _____

Note _____

_____

_____

Date _____Phone (   ) _____

Facility_____

Address _____

City _____ State _____ Zip_____

Requested by _____Dr. _____

Purpose _____

_____

Request copy of: ❏ Report　❏ X-rays　❏ Lab Results　❏ Other _____

Prepare for test: ❏ No　　❏ Yes _____

Note _____

_____

_____

Laboratory Work * X-Ray *(vertical sidebar tab)*

Laboratory Work * X-Ray Log

❏ **LABORATORY WORK**   ❏ **X-RAY**
(Best to use a separate page for each category.)

Date _____Phone (   )_____

Facility_____

Address _____

City _____ State _____ Zip_____

Requested by _____Dr. _____

Purpose _____

_____

Request copy of: ❏ Report   ❏ X-rays   ❏ Lab Results   ❏ Other _____

Prepare for test: ❏ No   ❏ Yes_____

Note _____

_____

_____

Date _____Phone (   )_____

Facility_____

Address _____

City _____ State _____ Zip_____

Requested by _____Dr. _____

Purpose _____

_____

Request copy of: ❏ Report   ❏ X-rays   ❏ Lab Results   ❏ Other _____

Prepare for test: ❏ No   ❏ Yes_____

Note _____

_____

_____

Laboratory Work * X-Ray Log

❏ **LABORATORY WORK**   ❏ **X-RAY**
(Best to use a separate page for each category.)

Date _____ Phone (   ) _____

Facility _____

Address _____

City _____ State _____ Zip_____

Requested by _____ Dr. _____

Purpose _____

_____

Request copy of: ❏ Report   ❏ X-rays   ❏ Lab Results   ❏ Other _____

Prepare for test: ❏ No   ❏ Yes _____

Note _____

_____

_____

Date _____ Phone (   ) _____

Facility _____

Address _____

City _____ State _____ Zip_____

Requested by _____ Dr. _____

Purpose _____

_____

Request copy of: ❏ Report   ❏ X-rays   ❏ Lab Results   ❏ Other _____

Prepare for test: ❏ No   ❏ Yes _____

Note _____

_____

_____

Laboratory Work * X-Ray

Laboratory Work * X-Ray Log

❏ **LABORATORY WORK**　❏ **X-RAY**
(Best to use a separate page for each category.)

Date _____ Phone (___) _____

Facility _____

Address _____

City _____ State _____ Zip _____

Requested by _____ Dr. _____

Purpose _____

_____

Request copy of: ❏ Report　❏ X-rays　❏ Lab Results　❏ Other _____

Prepare for test: ❏ No　❏ Yes _____

Note _____

_____

_____

_____

Date _____ Phone (___) _____

Facility _____

Address _____

City _____ State _____ Zip _____

Requested by _____ Dr. _____

Purpose _____

_____

Request copy of: ❏ Report　❏ X-rays　❏ Lab Results　❏ Other _____

Prepare for test: ❏ No　❏ Yes _____

Note _____

_____

_____

Laboratory Work * X-Ray

Laboratory Work * X-Ray Log

❑ **LABORATORY WORK**　　❑ **X-RAY**
(Best to use a separate page for each category.)

Date _____ Phone (_____) _____

Facility _____

Address _____

City _____ State _____ Zip_____

Requested by _____ Dr. _____

Purpose _____

_____

Request copy of: ❑ Report　❑ X-rays　❑ Lab Results　❑ Other _____

Prepare for test: ❑ No　　❑ Yes_____

Note _____

_____

_____

───

Date _____ Phone (_____) _____

Facility _____

Address _____

City _____ State _____ Zip_____

Requested by _____ Dr. _____

Purpose _____

_____

Request copy of: ❑ Report　❑ X-rays　❑ Lab Results　❑ Other _____

Prepare for test: ❑ No　　❑ Yes_____

Note _____

_____

_____

Laboratory Work * X-Ray

Laboratory Work * X-Ray Log

❏ **LABORATORY WORK**   ❏ **X-RAY**

(Best to use a separate page for each category.)

Date _____Phone (   )_____

Facility_____

Address _____

City _____ State _____ Zip_____

Requested by _____Dr. _____

Purpose _____

_____

Request copy of: ❏ Report ❏ X-rays ❏ Lab Results ❏ Other _____

Prepare for test: ❏ No ❏ Yes_____

Note_____

_____

_____

Date _____Phone (   )_____

Facility_____

Address _____

City _____ State _____ Zip_____

Requested by _____Dr. _____

Purpose _____

_____

Request copy of: ❏ Report ❏ X-rays ❏ Lab Results ❏ Other _____

Prepare for test: ❏ No ❏ Yes_____

Note_____

_____

_____

Laboratory Work * X-Ray Log

❏ **LABORATORY WORK**   ❏ **X-RAY**
(Best to use a separate page for each category.)

Date _____Phone (   )_____

Facility_____

Address _____

City _____ State _____ Zip_____

Requested by _____Dr. _____

Purpose _____

_____

Request copy of: ❏ Report   ❏ X-rays   ❏ Lab Results   ❏ Other _____

Prepare for test: ❏ No   ❏ Yes_____

Note _____

_____

_____

Date _____Phone (   )_____

Facility_____

Address _____

City _____ State _____ Zip_____

Requested by _____Dr. _____

Purpose _____

_____

Request copy of: ❏ Report   ❏ X-rays   ❏ Lab Results   ❏ Other _____

Prepare for test: ❏ No   ❏ Yes_____

Note _____

_____

_____

Laboratory Work * X-Ray

Immunization Log
Immunization Log * Shot Injection Log
Immunization Records * Shot Injection Records

Immunizations: These records will be needed throughout your lifetime.

Immunizations

Notes

Immunizations

Immunization Log

Place the month and year in the box. If you observe a reaction to the immunization complete the *'Immunization Record'* with the pertinent information needed to assist the physician. Also, mark the box with an *'R'* next to the date to know which immunization showed a reaction.

Booster *[Per physician recommendations]*

Chickenpox (VZV) *[Once at 1- 1 1/2 years]*

Diphtheria, Tetanus, Pertussis (DPT/Td) *[4 times at 0 - 1 1/2 years]*

Hepatitis B (HBV) *[3 times at 0 - 1 1/2 years]*

Measles, Mumps, Rubella (MMR) *[Once around 1 1/2 years]*

Polio (OPV) *[3 times in first year]*

Tuberculosis (TB Test) *[PRN]*

Other: Type _____

Continue on the back page if needed.

Note: Children and adults with special risk factors and/or allergies may require additional or alternative immunizations. Always discuss with your physician the risks involved with any immunization and treatment.

Immunization Log

You can record any shot treatment or immunization. Be sure to write on the *'Immunization Record'* (the next page) any problems or the reason for the treatment.

Other: Type _____

Other: Type _____

Other: Type _____

Other: Type _____

Other: Type _____

Other: Type _____

Other: Type _____

Other: Type _____

Other: Type _____

Immunizations

Immunization Records * Shot Injection Records

Date _____ Doctor / Clinic _____

Type _____

Reaction _____

Counteraction _____

Instructions _____

_____

_____

_____

Date _____ Doctor / Clinic _____

Type _____

Reaction _____

Counteraction _____

Instructions _____

_____

_____

_____

Date _____ Doctor / Clinic _____

Type _____

Reaction _____

Counteraction _____

Instructions _____

_____

_____

_____

Immunizations

Immunization Records * Shot Injection Records

Date _____ Doctor / Clinic _____

Type _____

Reaction _____

Counteraction _____

Instructions _____

_____

_____

_____

Date _____ Doctor / Clinic _____

Type _____

Reaction _____

Counteraction _____

Instructions _____

_____

_____

_____

Date _____ Doctor / Clinic _____

Type _____

Reaction _____

Counteraction _____

Instructions _____

_____

_____

_____

Immunizations

Immunization Records * Shot Injection Records

Date _____ Doctor / Clinic _____

Type _____

Reaction _____

Counteraction _____

Instructions _____

_____

_____

_____

Date _____ Doctor / Clinic _____

Type _____

Reaction _____

Counteraction _____

Instructions _____

_____

_____

_____

Date _____ Doctor / Clinic _____

Type _____

Reaction _____

Counteraction _____

Instructions _____

_____

_____

_____

Immunizations

Immunization Records ∗ Shot Injection Records

Date _____Doctor / Clinic_____

Type _____

Reaction_____

Counteraction _____

Instructions _____

_____

_____

_____

Date _____Doctor / Clinic_____

Type _____

Reaction_____

Counteraction _____

Instructions _____

_____

_____

_____

Date _____Doctor / Clinic_____

Type _____

Reaction_____

Counteraction _____

Instructions _____

_____

_____

_____

Immunizations

Immunization Records * Shot Injection Records

Date _____ Doctor / Clinic _____

Type _____

Reaction _____

Counteraction _____

Instructions _____

_____

_____

_____

Date _____ Doctor / Clinic _____

Type _____

Reaction _____

Counteraction _____

Instructions _____

_____

_____

_____

Date _____ Doctor / Clinic _____

Type _____

Reaction _____

Counteraction _____

Instructions _____

_____

_____

_____

Immunizations

Immunization Records ∗ Shot Injection Records

Date _____ Doctor / Clinic _____

Type _____

Reaction _____

Counteraction _____

Instructions _____

_____

_____

_____

Date _____ Doctor / Clinic _____

Type _____

Reaction _____

Counteraction _____

Instructions _____

_____

_____

_____

Date _____ Doctor / Clinic _____

Type _____

Reaction _____

Counteraction _____

Instructions _____

_____

_____

_____

Immunizations

Immunization Records ∗ Shot Injection Records

Date _____Doctor / Clinic _____

Type _____

Reaction _____

Counteraction _____

Instructions _____

_____

_____

_____

Date _____Doctor / Clinic _____

Type _____

Reaction _____

Counteraction _____

Instructions _____

_____

_____

_____

Date _____Doctor / Clinic _____

Type _____

Reaction _____

Counteraction _____

Instructions _____

_____

_____

_____

Immunizations

Immunization Records * Shot Injection Records

Date _____ Doctor / Clinic _____

Type _____

Reaction _____

Counteraction _____

Instructions _____

_____

_____

_____

Date _____ Doctor / Clinic _____

Type _____

Reaction _____

Counteraction _____

Instructions _____

_____

_____

_____

Date _____ Doctor / Clinic _____

Type _____

Reaction _____

Counteraction _____

Instructions _____

_____

_____

_____

Immunizations

Immunization Records * Shot Injection Records

Date _____Doctor / Clinic_____

Type _____

Reaction_____

Counteraction _____

Instructions _____

_____

_____

_____

Date _____Doctor / Clinic_____

Type _____

Reaction_____

Counteraction _____

Instructions _____

_____

_____

_____

Date _____Doctor / Clinic_____

Type _____

Reaction_____

Counteraction _____

Instructions _____

_____

_____

_____

Immunizations

Immunization Records * Shot Injection Records

Date _____ Doctor / Clinic _____

Type _____

Reaction _____

Counteraction _____

Instructions _____

_____

_____

_____

Date _____ Doctor / Clinic _____

Type _____

Reaction _____

Counteraction _____

Instructions _____

_____

_____

_____

Immunizations

Date _____ Doctor / Clinic _____

Type _____

Reaction _____

Counteraction _____

Instructions _____

_____

_____

_____

Academic Programs * Service Agencies

Academic Programs * Service Agencies: If you are utilizing the services of a special program, association or provider, it will be helpful to have the information available to share with your professional team. If this section is not needed, I would recommend removing it and saving it for another time.

Notes

Academic Programs * Service Agencies

❏ **ACADEMIC PROGRAMS** ❏ **SERVICE AGENCIES**

(Best to use a separate page for each category. Add the address and phone numbers in the address section. Also, collect business cards for easy reference.)

Date _____

School / Agency _____

Address _____

City _____ State _____ Zip_____

Phone (   )_____ (   )_____

Meeting with Teacher or (other) _____

Purpose _____

_____Preparation _____

❏ IEP   ❏ Funding   ❏ Other_____

NEXT APPOINTMENT: Date_____ Time _____

Summary _____

_____

Date _____

School / Agency _____ _____

Address _____

City _____ State _____ Zip_____

Phone (   )_____ (   )_____

Meeting with Teacher or (other) _____

Purpose _____

_____Preparation _____

❏ IEP   ❏ Funding   ❏ Other_____

NEXT APPOINTMENT: Date_____ Time _____

Summary _____

_____

Academic Programs * Service Agencies

❑ **ACADEMIC PROGRAMS**   ❑ **SERVICE AGENCIES**

(Best to use a separate page for each category. Add the address and phone numbers in the address section. Also, collect business cards for easy reference.)

Date _____

School / Agency _____

Address _____

City _____ State _____ Zip_____

Phone (   )_____ (   )_____

Meeting with Teacher or (other) _____

Purpose _____

_____Preparation _____

❑ IEP   ❑ Funding   ❑ Other_____

NEXT APPOINTMENT: Date_____ Time _____

Summary _____

_____

Date _____

School / Agency _____

Address _____

City _____ State _____ Zip_____

Phone (   )_____ (   )_____

Meeting with Teacher or (other) _____

Purpose _____

_____Preparation _____

❑ IEP   ❑ Funding   ❑ Other_____

NEXT APPOINTMENT: Date_____ Time _____

Summary _____

_____

Academic Programs Service Agencies

Academic Programs * Service Agencies

❏ **ACADEMIC PROGRAMS**   ❏ **SERVICE AGENCIES**

(Best to use a separate page for each category. Add the address and phone numbers in the address section. Also, collect business cards for easy reference.)

Date _____

School / Agency _____

Address _____

City _____ State _____ Zip_____

Phone (   )_____ (   )_____

Meeting with Teacher or (other)_____

Purpose _____

_____Preparation _____

❏ IEP   ❏ Funding   ❏ Other_____

NEXT APPOINTMENT: Date_____ Time _____

Summary _____

_____

Date _____

School / Agency _____

Address _____

City _____ State _____ Zip_____

Phone (   )_____ (   )_____

Meeting with Teacher or (other)_____

Purpose _____

_____Preparation _____

❏ IEP   ❏ Funding   ❏ Other_____

NEXT APPOINTMENT: Date_____ Time _____

Summary _____

_____

Academic Programs * Service Agencies

❑ **ACADEMIC PROGRAMS**   ❑ **SERVICE AGENCIES**

(Best to use a separate page for each category. Add the address and phone numbers in the address section. Also, collect business cards for easy reference.)

Date _____

School / Agency _____

Address _____

City _____ State _____ Zip_____

Phone (   )_____ (   )_____

Meeting with Teacher or (other) _____

Purpose _____

_____Preparation _____

❑ IEP   ❑ Funding   ❑ Other_____

NEXT APPOINTMENT: Date_____ Time _____

Summary _____

_____

Date _____

School / Agency _____

Address _____

City _____ State _____ Zip_____

Phone (   )_____ (   )_____

Meeting with Teacher or (other) _____

Purpose _____

_____Preparation _____

❑ IEP   ❑ Funding   ❑ Other_____

NEXT APPOINTMENT: Date_____ Time _____

Summary _____

_____

**Academic Programs
Service Agencies**

Academic Programs * Service Agencies

❏ **ACADEMIC PROGRAMS** ❏ **SERVICE AGENCIES**

(Best to use a separate page for each category. Add the address and phone numbers in the address section. Also, collect business cards for easy reference.)

Date _____

School / Agency _____

Address _____

City _____ State _____ Zip_____

Phone ( ) _____ ( ) _____

Meeting with Teacher or (other) _____

Purpose _____

_____Preparation _____

❏ IEP ❏ Funding ❏ Other_____

NEXT APPOINTMENT: Date_____ Time _____

Summary _____

_____

Date _____

School / Agency _____

Address _____

City _____ State _____ Zip_____

Phone ( ) _____ ( ) _____

Meeting with Teacher or (other) _____

Purpose _____

_____Preparation _____

❏ IEP ❏ Funding ❏ Other_____

NEXT APPOINTMENT: Date_____ Time _____

Summary _____

_____

Academic Programs ∗ Service Agencies

❏ **ACADEMIC PROGRAMS**   ❏ **SERVICE AGENCIES**

(Best to use a separate page for each category. Add the address and phone numbers in the address section. Also, collect business cards for easy reference.)

Date _____

School / Agency _____

Address _____

City _____ State _____ Zip _____

Phone (____) _____ (____) _____

Meeting with Teacher or (other) _____

Purpose _____

_____Preparation _____

❏ IEP ❏ Funding ❏ Other_____

NEXT APPOINTMENT: Date_____ Time _____

Summary _____

_____

Date _____

School / Agency _____

Address _____

City _____ State _____ Zip _____

Phone (____) _____ (____) _____

Meeting with Teacher or (other) _____

Purpose _____

_____Preparation _____

❏ IEP ❏ Funding ❏ Other_____

NEXT APPOINTMENT: Date_____ Time _____

Summary _____

_____

Academic Programs Service Agencies

Names & Addresses Index

Names and Addresses: Keep the phone numbers and addresses of any one who is assisting you with your medical / dental health care.

Notes

Names & Addresses Index

Listing from _____ to _____

❑ **DOCTOR**　❑ **HOSPITAL**　❑ **SERVICE**　❑ **AGENCY**　❑ **THERAPIST**

(You may want to group by discipline or service per page.)

Name _____ Phone _____
Specialty Field _____ Fax _____
Nurse _____ Other_____
Hospital _____ Email_____
Clinic / Dept. _____
Address _____ Ste/Room _____
City _____ State _____ Zip_____
Note _____

Name _____ Phone _____
Specialty Field _____ Fax _____
Nurse _____ Other_____
Hospital _____ Email_____
Clinic / Dept. _____
Address _____ Ste/Room _____
City _____ State _____ Zip_____
Note _____

Name _____ Phone _____
Specialty Field _____ Fax _____
Nurse _____ Other_____
Hospital _____ Email_____
Clinic / Dept. _____
Address _____ Ste/Room _____
City _____ State _____ Zip_____
Note _____

Name _____ Phone _____
Specialty Field _____ Fax _____
Nurse _____ Other_____
Hospital _____ Email_____
Clinic / Dept. _____
Address _____ Ste/Room _____
City _____ State _____ Zip_____
Note _____

Names & Addresses Index

Listing from _____ to _____

❏ DOCTOR   ❏ HOSPITAL   ❏ SERVICE   ❏ AGENCY   ❏ THERAPIST

(You may want to group by discipline or service per page.)

Name _____ Phone _____

Specialty Field _____ Fax _____

Nurse _____ Other _____

Hospital _____ Email _____

Clinic / Dept. _____

Address _____ Ste/Room _____

City _____ State _____ Zip _____

Note _____

Name _____ Phone _____

Specialty Field _____ Fax _____

Nurse _____ Other _____

Hospital _____ Email _____

Clinic / Dept. _____

Address _____ Ste/Room _____

City _____ State _____ Zip _____

Note _____

Name _____ Phone _____

Specialty Field _____ Fax _____

Nurse _____ Other _____

Hospital _____ Email _____

Clinic / Dept. _____

Address _____ Ste/Room _____

City _____ State _____ Zip _____

Note _____

Name _____ Phone _____

Specialty Field _____ Fax _____

Nurse _____ Other _____

Hospital _____ Email _____

Clinic / Dept. _____

Address _____ Ste/Room _____

City _____ State _____ Zip _____

Note _____

Names & Addresses Index

Listing from _____ to _____

❏ **DOCTOR**   ❏ **HOSPITAL**   ❏ **SERVICE**   ❏ **AGENCY**   ❏ **THERAPIST**

(You may want to group by discipline or service per page.)

Name _____ Phone _____

Specialty Field _____ Fax _____

Nurse _____ Other _____

Hospital _____ Email _____

Clinic / Dept. _____

Address _____ Ste/Room _____

City _____ State _____ Zip _____

Note _____

Name _____ Phone _____

Specialty Field _____ Fax _____

Nurse _____ Other _____

Hospital _____ Email _____

Clinic / Dept. _____

Address _____ Ste/Room _____

City _____ State _____ Zip _____

Note _____

Name _____ Phone _____

Specialty Field _____ Fax _____

Nurse _____ Other _____

Hospital _____ Email _____

Clinic / Dept. _____

Address _____ Ste/Room _____

City _____ State _____ Zip _____

Note _____

Name _____ Phone _____

Specialty Field _____ Fax _____

Nurse _____ Other _____

Hospital _____ Email _____

Clinic / Dept. _____

Address _____ Ste/Room _____

City _____ State _____ Zip _____

Note _____

Names & Addresses Index

Listing from _____ to _____

❏ **DOCTOR**   ❏ **HOSPITAL**   ❏ **SERVICE**   ❏ **AGENCY**   ❏ **THERAPIST**

(You may want to group by discipline or service per page.)

Name _____   Phone _____
Specialty Field _____   Fax _____
Nurse _____   Other_____
Hospital _____   Email_____
Clinic / Dept. _____
Address _____   Ste/Room _____
City _____State _____   Zip_____
Note _____

Name _____   Phone _____
Specialty Field _____   Fax _____
Nurse _____   Other_____
Hospital _____   Email_____
Clinic / Dept. _____
Address _____   Ste/Room _____
City _____State _____   Zip_____
Note _____

Name _____   Phone _____
Specialty Field _____   Fax _____
Nurse _____   Other_____
Hospital _____   Email_____
Clinic / Dept. _____
Address _____   Ste/Room _____
City _____State _____   Zip_____
Note _____

Name _____   Phone _____
Specialty Field _____   Fax _____
Nurse _____   Other_____
Hospital _____   Email_____
Clinic / Dept. _____
Address _____   Ste/Room _____
City _____State _____   Zip_____
Note _____

Names & Addresses Index

Listing from _____ to _____

❏ DOCTOR ❏ HOSPITAL ❏ SERVICE ❏ AGENCY ❏ THERAPIST

(You may want to group by discipline or service per page.)

Name _____ Phone _____

Specialty Field _____ Fax _____

Nurse _____ Other _____

Hospital _____ Email _____

Clinic / Dept. _____

Address _____ Ste/Room _____

City _____ State _____ Zip_____

Note _____

Name _____ Phone _____

Specialty Field _____ Fax _____

Nurse _____ Other _____

Hospital _____ Email _____

Clinic / Dept. _____

Address _____ Ste/Room _____

City _____ State _____ Zip_____

Note _____

Name _____ Phone _____

Specialty Field _____ Fax _____

Nurse _____ Other _____

Hospital _____ Email _____

Clinic / Dept. _____

Address _____ Ste/Room _____

City _____ State _____ Zip_____

Note _____

Name _____ Phone _____

Specialty Field _____ Fax _____

Nurse _____ Other _____

Hospital _____ Email _____

Clinic / Dept. _____

Address _____ Ste/Room _____

City _____ State _____ Zip_____

Note _____

Names & Addresses Index

Listing from _____ to _____

❏ **DOCTOR**   ❏ **HOSPITAL**   ❏ **SERVICE**   ❏ **AGENCY**   ❏ **THERAPIST**

(You may want to group by discipline or service per page.)

Name _____ Phone _____
Specialty Field _____ Fax _____
Nurse _____ Other_____
Hospital _____ Email_____
Clinic / Dept. _____
Address _____ Ste/Room _____
City _____State _____ Zip_____
Note _____

Name _____ Phone _____
Specialty Field _____ Fax _____
Nurse _____ Other_____
Hospital _____ Email_____
Clinic / Dept. _____
Address _____ Ste/Room _____
City _____State _____ Zip_____
Note _____

Name _____ Phone _____
Specialty Field _____ Fax _____
Nurse _____ Other_____
Hospital _____ Email_____
Clinic / Dept. _____
Address _____ Ste/Room _____
City _____State _____ Zip_____
Note _____

Name _____ Phone _____
Specialty Field _____ Fax _____
Nurse _____ Other_____
Hospital _____ Email_____
Clinic / Dept. _____
Address _____ Ste/Room _____
City _____State _____ Zip_____
Note _____

Names & Addresses Index

Listing from _____ to _____

❏ **DOCTOR**   ❏ **HOSPITAL**   ❏ **SERVICE**   ❏ **AGENCY**   ❏ **THERAPIST**

(You may want to group by discipline or service per page.)

Name _____ Phone _____
Specialty Field _____ Fax _____
Nurse _____ Other_____
Hospital _____ Email_____
Clinic / Dept. _____
Address _____ Ste/Room _____
City _____ State _____ Zip_____
Note _____

Name _____ Phone _____
Specialty Field _____ Fax _____
Nurse _____ Other_____
Hospital _____ Email_____
Clinic / Dept. _____
Address _____ Ste/Room _____
City _____ State _____ Zip_____
Note _____

Name _____ Phone _____
Specialty Field _____ Fax _____
Nurse _____ Other_____
Hospital _____ Email_____
Clinic / Dept. _____
Address _____ Ste/Room _____
City _____ State _____ Zip_____
Note _____

Name _____ Phone _____
Specialty Field _____ Fax _____
Nurse _____ Other_____
Hospital _____ Email_____
Clinic / Dept. _____
Address _____ Ste/Room _____
City _____ State _____ Zip_____
Note _____

Names & Addresses Index

Listing from _____ to _____

☐ DOCTOR   ☐ HOSPITAL   ☐ SERVICE   ☐ AGENCY   ☐ THERAPIST

(You may want to group by discipline or service per page.)

Name _____ Phone _____
Specialty Field _____ Fax _____
Nurse _____ Other _____
Hospital _____ Email _____
Clinic / Dept. _____
Address _____ Ste/Room _____
City _____ State _____ Zip _____
Note _____

Name _____ Phone _____
Specialty Field _____ Fax _____
Nurse _____ Other _____
Hospital _____ Email _____
Clinic / Dept. _____
Address _____ Ste/Room _____
City _____ State _____ Zip _____
Note _____

Name _____ Phone _____
Specialty Field _____ Fax _____
Nurse _____ Other _____
Hospital _____ Email _____
Clinic / Dept. _____
Address _____ Ste/Room _____
City _____ State _____ Zip _____
Note _____

Name _____ Phone _____
Specialty Field _____ Fax _____
Nurse _____ Other _____
Hospital _____ Email _____
Clinic / Dept. _____
Address _____ Ste/Room _____
City _____ State _____ Zip _____
Note _____

Names & Addresses Index

Listing from _____ to _____

❏ **DOCTOR** ❏ **HOSPITAL** ❏ **SERVICE** ❏ **AGENCY** ❏ **THERAPIST**

(You may want to group by discipline or service per page.)

Name _____ Phone _____

Specialty Field _____ Fax _____

Nurse _____ Other _____

Hospital _____ Email _____

Clinic / Dept. _____

Address _____ Ste/Room _____

City _____ State _____ Zip_____

Note _____

Name _____ Phone _____

Specialty Field _____ Fax _____

Nurse _____ Other _____

Hospital _____ Email _____

Clinic / Dept. _____

Address _____ Ste/Room _____

City _____ State _____ Zip_____

Note _____

Name _____ Phone _____

Specialty Field _____ Fax _____

Nurse _____ Other _____

Hospital _____ Email _____

Clinic / Dept. _____

Address _____ Ste/Room _____

City _____ State _____ Zip_____

Note _____

Name _____ Phone _____

Specialty Field _____ Fax _____

Nurse _____ Other _____

Hospital _____ Email _____

Clinic / Dept. _____

Address _____ Ste/Room _____

City _____ State _____ Zip_____

Note _____

Names & Addresses Index

Listing from _____ to _____

❑ **DOCTOR**   ❑ **HOSPITAL**   ❑ **SERVICE**   ❑ **AGENCY**   ❑ **THERAPIST**

(You may want to group by discipline or service per page.)

Name _____ Phone _____

Specialty Field _____ Fax _____

Nurse _____ Other_____

Hospital _____ Email_____

Clinic / Dept. _____

Address _____ Ste/Room _____

City _____State _____ Zip_____

Note _____

Name _____ Phone _____

Specialty Field _____ Fax _____

Nurse _____ Other_____

Hospital _____ Email_____

Clinic / Dept. _____

Address _____ Ste/Room _____

City _____State _____ Zip_____

Note _____

Name _____ Phone _____

Specialty Field _____ Fax _____

Nurse _____ Other_____

Hospital _____ Email_____

Clinic / Dept. _____

Address _____ Ste/Room _____

City _____State _____ Zip_____

Note _____

Name _____ Phone _____

Specialty Field _____ Fax _____

Nurse _____ Other_____

Hospital _____ Email_____

Clinic / Dept. _____

Address _____ Ste/Room _____

City _____State _____ Zip_____

Note _____

Names & Addresses Index

Listing from _____ to _____

☐ **DOCTOR**   ☐ **HOSPITAL**   ☐ **SERVICE**   ☐ **AGENCY**   ☐ **THERAPIST**

(You may want to group by discipline or service per page.)

Name _____ Phone _____

Specialty Field _____ Fax _____

Nurse _____ Other _____

Hospital _____ Email _____

Clinic / Dept. _____

Address _____ Ste/Room _____

City _____ State _____ Zip _____

Note _____

Name _____ Phone _____

Specialty Field _____ Fax _____

Nurse _____ Other _____

Hospital _____ Email _____

Clinic / Dept. _____

Address _____ Ste/Room _____

City _____ State _____ Zip _____

Note _____

Name _____ Phone _____

Specialty Field _____ Fax _____

Nurse _____ Other _____

Hospital _____ Email _____

Clinic / Dept. _____

Address _____ Ste/Room _____

City _____ State _____ Zip _____

Note _____

Name _____ Phone _____

Specialty Field _____ Fax _____

Nurse _____ Other _____

Hospital _____ Email _____

Clinic / Dept. _____

Address _____ Ste/Room _____

City _____ State _____ Zip _____

Note _____

Names & Addresses Index

Listing from _____ to _____

❑ DOCTOR   ❑ HOSPITAL   ❑ SERVICE   ❑ AGENCY   ❑ THERAPIST

(You may want to group by discipline or service per page.)

Name _____ Phone _____

Specialty Field _____ Fax _____

Nurse _____ Other _____

Hospital _____ Email _____

Clinic / Dept. _____

Address _____ Ste/Room _____

City _____ State _____ Zip _____

Note _____

Name _____ Phone _____

Specialty Field _____ Fax _____

Nurse _____ Other _____

Hospital _____ Email _____

Clinic / Dept. _____

Address _____ Ste/Room _____

City _____ State _____ Zip _____

Note _____

Name _____ Phone _____

Specialty Field _____ Fax _____

Nurse _____ Other _____

Hospital _____ Email _____

Clinic / Dept. _____

Address _____ Ste/Room _____

City _____ State _____ Zip _____

Note _____

Name _____ Phone _____

Specialty Field _____ Fax _____

Nurse _____ Other _____

Hospital _____ Email _____

Clinic / Dept. _____

Address _____ Ste/Room _____

City _____ State _____ Zip _____

Note _____

Names & Addresses Index

Listing from _____ to _____

❏ DOCTOR   ❏ HOSPITAL   ❏ SERVICE   ❏ AGENCY   ❏ THERAPIST

(You may want to group by discipline or service per page.)

Name _____ Phone _____
Specialty Field _____ Fax _____
Nurse _____ Other _____
Hospital _____ Email _____
Clinic / Dept. _____
Address _____ Ste/Room _____
City _____ State _____ Zip _____
Note _____

Name _____ Phone _____
Specialty Field _____ Fax _____
Nurse _____ Other _____
Hospital _____ Email _____
Clinic / Dept. _____
Address _____ Ste/Room _____
City _____ State _____ Zip _____
Note _____

Name _____ Phone _____
Specialty Field _____ Fax _____
Nurse _____ Other _____
Hospital _____ Email _____
Clinic / Dept. _____
Address _____ Ste/Room _____
City _____ State _____ Zip _____
Note _____

Name _____ Phone _____
Specialty Field _____ Fax _____
Nurse _____ Other _____
Hospital _____ Email _____
Clinic / Dept. _____
Address _____ Ste/Room _____
City _____ State _____ Zip _____
Note _____

Names & Addresses Index

Listing from _____ to _____

❏ DOCTOR   ❏ HOSPITAL   ❏ SERVICE   ❏ AGENCY   ❏ THERAPIST

(You may want to group by discipline or service per page.)

Name _____ Phone _____

Specialty Field _____ Fax _____

Nurse _____ Other_____

Hospital _____ Email_____

Clinic / Dept. _____

Address _____ Ste/Room _____

City _____State _____ Zip_____

Note _____

Name _____ Phone _____

Specialty Field _____ Fax _____

Nurse _____ Other_____

Hospital _____ Email_____

Clinic / Dept. _____

Address _____ Ste/Room _____

City _____State _____ Zip_____

Note _____

Name _____ Phone _____

Specialty Field _____ Fax _____

Nurse _____ Other_____

Hospital _____ Email_____

Clinic / Dept. _____

Address _____ Ste/Room _____

City _____State _____ Zip_____

Note _____

Name _____ Phone _____

Specialty Field _____ Fax _____

Nurse _____ Other_____

Hospital _____ Email_____

Clinic / Dept. _____

Address _____ Ste/Room _____

City _____State _____ Zip_____

Note _____

Names & Addresses Index

Listing from _____ to _____

❑ DOCTOR   ❑ HOSPITAL   ❑ SERVICE   ❑ AGENCY   ❑ THERAPIST

(You may want to group by discipline or service per page.)

Name _____ Phone _____
Specialty Field _____ Fax _____
Nurse _____ Other_____
Hospital _____ Email_____
Clinic / Dept. _____
Address _____ Ste/Room _____
City _____State _____ Zip_____
Note _____

Name _____ Phone _____
Specialty Field _____ Fax _____
Nurse _____ Other_____
Hospital _____ Email_____
Clinic / Dept. _____
Address _____ Ste/Room _____
City _____State _____ Zip_____
Note _____

Name _____ Phone _____
Specialty Field _____ Fax _____
Nurse _____ Other_____
Hospital _____ Email_____
Clinic / Dept. _____
Address _____ Ste/Room _____
City _____State _____ Zip_____
Note _____

Name _____ Phone _____
Specialty Field _____ Fax _____
Nurse _____ Other_____
Hospital _____ Email_____
Clinic / Dept. _____
Address _____ Ste/Room _____
City _____State _____ Zip_____
Note _____

Names & Addresses Index

Listing from _____ to _____

❏ DOCTOR   ❏ HOSPITAL   ❏ SERVICE   ❏ AGENCY   ❏ THERAPIST

(You may want to group by discipline or service per page.)

Name _____ Phone _____

Specialty Field _____ Fax _____

Nurse _____ Other_____

Hospital _____ Email_____

Clinic / Dept. _____

Address _____ Ste/Room _____

City _____State _____ Zip_____

Note _____

Name _____ Phone _____

Specialty Field _____ Fax _____

Nurse _____ Other_____

Hospital _____ Email_____

Clinic / Dept. _____

Address _____ Ste/Room _____

City _____State _____ Zip_____

Note _____

Name _____ Phone _____

Specialty Field _____ Fax _____

Nurse _____ Other_____

Hospital _____ Email_____

Clinic / Dept. _____

Address _____ Ste/Room _____

City _____State _____ Zip_____

Note _____

Name _____ Phone _____

Specialty Field _____ Fax _____

Nurse _____ Other_____

Hospital _____ Email_____

Clinic / Dept. _____

Address _____ Ste/Room _____

City _____State _____ Zip_____

Note _____

Names & Addresses Index

Listing from _____ to _____

❏ **DOCTOR**   ❏ **HOSPITAL**   ❏ **SERVICE**   ❏ **AGENCY**   ❏ **THERAPIST**

(You may want to group by discipline or service per page.)

Name _____ Phone _____

Specialty Field _____ Fax _____

Nurse _____ Other _____

Hospital _____ Email _____

Clinic / Dept. _____

Address _____ Ste/Room _____

City _____ State _____ Zip_____

Note _____

Name _____ Phone _____

Specialty Field _____ Fax _____

Nurse _____ Other _____

Hospital _____ Email _____

Clinic / Dept. _____

Address _____ Ste/Room _____

City _____ State _____ Zip_____

Note _____

Name _____ Phone _____

Specialty Field _____ Fax _____

Nurse _____ Other _____

Hospital _____ Email _____

Clinic / Dept. _____

Address _____ Ste/Room _____

City _____ State _____ Zip_____

Note _____

Name _____ Phone _____

Specialty Field _____ Fax _____

Nurse _____ Other _____

Hospital _____ Email _____

Clinic / Dept. _____

Address _____ Ste/Room _____

City _____ State _____ Zip_____

Note _____

Names & Addresses Index

Listing from _____ to _____

❏ DOCTOR   ❏ HOSPITAL   ❏ SERVICE   ❏ AGENCY   ❏ THERAPIST

(You may want to group by discipline or service per page.)

Name _____ Phone _____

Specialty Field _____ Fax _____

Nurse _____ Other_____

Hospital _____ Email_____

Clinic / Dept. _____

Address _____ Ste/Room _____

City _____State _____ Zip_____

Note _____

Name _____ Phone _____

Specialty Field _____ Fax _____

Nurse _____ Other_____

Hospital _____ Email_____

Clinic / Dept. _____

Address _____ Ste/Room _____

City _____State _____ Zip_____

Note _____

Name _____ Phone _____

Specialty Field _____ Fax _____

Nurse _____ Other_____

Hospital _____ Email_____

Clinic / Dept. _____

Address _____ Ste/Room _____

City _____State _____ Zip_____

Note _____

Name _____ Phone _____

Specialty Field _____ Fax _____

Nurse _____ Other_____

Hospital _____ Email_____

Clinic / Dept. _____

Address _____ Ste/Room _____

City _____State _____ Zip_____

Note _____

Names & Addresses Index

Listing from _____ to _____

❏ **DOCTOR**   ❏ **HOSPITAL**   ❏ **SERVICE**   ❏ **AGENCY**   ❏ **THERAPIST**

(You may want to group by discipline or service per page.)

Name _____ Phone _____
Specialty Field _____ Fax _____
Nurse _____ Other _____
Hospital _____ Email _____
Clinic / Dept. _____
Address _____ Ste/Room _____
City _____ State _____ Zip _____
Note _____

Name _____ Phone _____
Specialty Field _____ Fax _____
Nurse _____ Other _____
Hospital _____ Email _____
Clinic / Dept. _____
Address _____ Ste/Room _____
City _____ State _____ Zip _____
Note _____

Name _____ Phone _____
Specialty Field _____ Fax _____
Nurse _____ Other _____
Hospital _____ Email _____
Clinic / Dept. _____
Address _____ Ste/Room _____
City _____ State _____ Zip _____
Note _____

Name _____ Phone _____
Specialty Field _____ Fax _____
Nurse _____ Other _____
Hospital _____ Email _____
Clinic / Dept. _____
Address _____ Ste/Room _____
City _____ State _____ Zip _____
Note _____

Names & Addresses

Names & Addresses Index

Listing from _____ to _____

❏ DOCTOR ❏ HOSPITAL ❏ SERVICE ❏ AGENCY ❏ THERAPIST

(You may want to group by discipline or service per page.)

Name _____ Phone _____
Specialty Field _____ Fax _____
Nurse _____ Other _____
Hospital _____ Email _____
Clinic / Dept. _____
Address _____ Ste/Room _____
City _____ State _____ Zip _____
Note _____

Name _____ Phone _____
Specialty Field _____ Fax _____
Nurse _____ Other _____
Hospital _____ Email _____
Clinic / Dept. _____
Address _____ Ste/Room _____
City _____ State _____ Zip _____
Note _____

Name _____ Phone _____
Specialty Field _____ Fax _____
Nurse _____ Other _____
Hospital _____ Email _____
Clinic / Dept. _____
Address _____ Ste/Room _____
City _____ State _____ Zip _____
Note _____

Name _____ Phone _____
Specialty Field _____ Fax _____
Nurse _____ Other _____
Hospital _____ Email _____
Clinic / Dept. _____
Address _____ Ste/Room _____
City _____ State _____ Zip _____
Note _____

Names & Addresses Index

Listing from _____ to _____

❏ **DOCTOR**　❏ **HOSPITAL**　❏ **SERVICE**　❏ **AGENCY**　❏ **THERAPIST**

(You may want to group by discipline or service per page.)

Name _____ Phone _____

Specialty Field _____ Fax _____

Nurse _____ Other _____

Hospital _____ Email _____

Clinic / Dept. _____

Address _____ Ste/Room _____

City _____ State _____ Zip_____

Note _____

Name _____ Phone _____

Specialty Field _____ Fax _____

Nurse _____ Other _____

Hospital _____ Email _____

Clinic / Dept. _____

Address _____ Ste/Room _____

City _____ State _____ Zip_____

Note _____

Name _____ Phone _____

Specialty Field _____ Fax _____

Nurse _____ Other _____

Hospital _____ Email _____

Clinic / Dept. _____

Address _____ Ste/Room _____

City _____ State _____ Zip_____

Note _____

Name _____ Phone _____

Specialty Field _____ Fax _____

Nurse _____ Other _____

Hospital _____ Email _____

Clinic / Dept. _____

Address _____ Ste/Room _____

City _____ State _____ Zip_____

Note _____

Names & Addresses Index

Listing from _____ to _____

❑ **DOCTOR**   ❑ **HOSPITAL**   ❑ **SERVICE**   ❑ **AGENCY**   ❑ **THERAPIST**

(You may want to group by discipline or service per page.)

Name _____ Phone _____

Specialty Field _____ Fax _____

Nurse _____ Other_____

Hospital _____ Email_____

Clinic / Dept. _____

Address _____ Ste/Room _____

City _____State _____ Zip_____

Note _____

Name _____ Phone _____

Specialty Field _____ Fax _____

Nurse _____ Other_____

Hospital _____ Email_____

Clinic / Dept. _____

Address _____ Ste/Room _____

City _____State _____ Zip_____

Note _____

Name _____ Phone _____

Specialty Field _____ Fax _____

Nurse _____ Other_____

Hospital _____ Email_____

Clinic / Dept. _____

Address _____ Ste/Room _____

City _____State _____ Zip_____

Note _____

Name _____ Phone _____

Specialty Field _____ Fax _____

Nurse _____ Other_____

Hospital _____ Email_____

Clinic / Dept. _____

Address _____ Ste/Room _____

City _____State _____ Zip_____

Note _____

Names & Addresses Index

Listing from _____ to _____

❏ **DOCTOR**   ❏ **HOSPITAL**   ❏ **SERVICE**   ❏ **AGENCY**   ❏ **THERAPIST**
(You may want to group by discipline or service per page.)

Name _____ Phone _____
Specialty Field _____ Fax _____
Nurse _____ Other_____
Hospital _____ Email_____
Clinic / Dept._____
Address _____ Ste/Room _____
City _____State _____ Zip_____
Note _____

Name _____ Phone _____
Specialty Field _____ Fax _____
Nurse _____ Other_____
Hospital _____ Email_____
Clinic / Dept._____
Address _____ Ste/Room _____
City _____State _____ Zip_____
Note _____

Name _____ Phone _____
Specialty Field _____ Fax _____
Nurse _____ Other_____
Hospital _____ Email_____
Clinic / Dept._____
Address _____ Ste/Room _____
City _____State _____ Zip_____
Note _____

Name _____ Phone _____
Specialty Field _____ Fax _____
Nurse _____ Other_____
Hospital _____ Email_____
Clinic / Dept._____
Address _____ Ste/Room _____
City _____State _____ Zip_____
Note _____

Names & Addresses Index

Listing from _____ to _____

❑ DOCTOR ❑ HOSPITAL ❑ SERVICE ❑ AGENCY ❑ THERAPIST

(You may want to group by discipline or service per page.)

Name _____ Phone _____

Specialty Field _____ Fax _____

Nurse _____ Other _____

Hospital _____ Email _____

Clinic / Dept. _____

Address _____ Ste/Room _____

City _____ State _____ Zip _____

Note _____

Name _____ Phone _____

Specialty Field _____ Fax _____

Nurse _____ Other _____

Hospital _____ Email _____

Clinic / Dept. _____

Address _____ Ste/Room _____

City _____ State _____ Zip _____

Note _____

Name _____ Phone _____

Specialty Field _____ Fax _____

Nurse _____ Other _____

Hospital _____ Email _____

Clinic / Dept. _____

Address _____ Ste/Room _____

City _____ State _____ Zip _____

Note _____

Name _____ Phone _____

Specialty Field _____ Fax _____

Nurse _____ Other _____

Hospital _____ Email _____

Clinic / Dept. _____

Address _____ Ste/Room _____

City _____ State _____ Zip _____

Note _____

Names & Addresses Index

Listing from _____ to _____

❑ **DOCTOR**   ❑ **HOSPITAL**   ❑ **SERVICE**   ❑ **AGENCY**   ❑ **THERAPIST**

(You may want to group by discipline or service per page.)

Name _____ Phone _____

Specialty Field _____ Fax _____

Nurse _____ Other _____

Hospital _____ Email _____

Clinic / Dept. _____

Address _____ Ste/Room _____

City _____ State _____ Zip_____

Note _____

Name _____ Phone _____

Specialty Field _____ Fax _____

Nurse _____ Other _____

Hospital _____ Email _____

Clinic / Dept. _____

Address _____ Ste/Room _____

City _____ State _____ Zip_____

Note _____

Name _____ Phone _____

Specialty Field _____ Fax _____

Nurse _____ Other _____

Hospital _____ Email _____

Clinic / Dept. _____

Address _____ Ste/Room _____

City _____ State _____ Zip_____

Note _____

Name _____ Phone _____

Specialty Field _____ Fax _____

Nurse _____ Other _____

Hospital _____ Email _____

Clinic / Dept. _____

Address _____ Ste/Room _____

City _____ State _____ Zip_____

Note _____

Names & Addresses

Names & Addresses Index

Listing from _____ to _____

❑ DOCTOR ❑ HOSPITAL ❑ SERVICE ❑ AGENCY ❑ THERAPIST
(You may want to group by discipline or service per page.)

Name _____ Phone _____
Specialty Field _____ Fax _____
Nurse _____ Other_____
Hospital _____ Email_____
Clinic / Dept. _____
Address _____ Ste/Room _____
City _____ State _____ Zip_____
Note _____

Name _____ Phone _____
Specialty Field _____ Fax _____
Nurse _____ Other_____
Hospital _____ Email_____
Clinic / Dept. _____
Address _____ Ste/Room _____
City _____ State _____ Zip_____
Note _____

Name _____ Phone _____
Specialty Field _____ Fax _____
Nurse _____ Other_____
Hospital _____ Email_____
Clinic / Dept. _____
Address _____ Ste/Room _____
City _____ State _____ Zip_____
Note _____

Name _____ Phone _____
Specialty Field _____ Fax _____
Nurse _____ Other_____
Hospital _____ Email_____
Clinic / Dept. _____
Address _____ Ste/Room _____
City _____ State _____ Zip_____
Note _____

© 2008 Life Cycles Publishing, Inc. All Rights Reserved.

244

REORDER FORM

For more information on additional sections, and supplies please send the attached card or check my web site at www.lifecyclespublishing.com.

Name _____

Company _____

Address _____ Apt/Ste. _____

City _____State _____ Zip_____ Country _____

Phone ( )_____ Ext_____

Fax ( ) _____

E-mail _____

I am interested in the following

❑ Additional books

❑ Additional sections

❑ Protective covers

❑ Other: _____

❑ My company / medical facility would like to be a sponsor, please call.

❑ I am arranging a meeting and would like to invite you to participate.

Location _____

Topic_____

Date _____ Time _____

Mail to: **Life Cycles Publishing, Inc.**

P.O. Box 3556

Fremont, CA 94539-0335

Complete your information, cut along dotted lines, fold and place into your wallet.

Personal Emergency Card

Name _____

Address _____ Apt. _____

City/State/Zip _____ Country _____

Phone (___) _____ Fax (___) _____

Email _____

Physician _____

Dr. Phone # (___) _____

Emergency Contact _____ State ____ Zip ____

Phone # (___) _____

Medications

	Type	Dose	Frequency
1.			
2.			
3.			
4.			
5.			
6.			
7.			

Personal Emergency Card

Name _____

Address _____ Apt. _____

City/State/Zip _____ Country _____

Phone (___) _____ Fax (___) _____

Email _____

Physician _____

Dr. Phone # (___) _____

Emergency Contact _____ State ____ Zip ____

Phone # (___) _____

Medications

	Type	Dose	Frequency
1.			
2.			
3.			
4.			
5.			
6.			
7.			

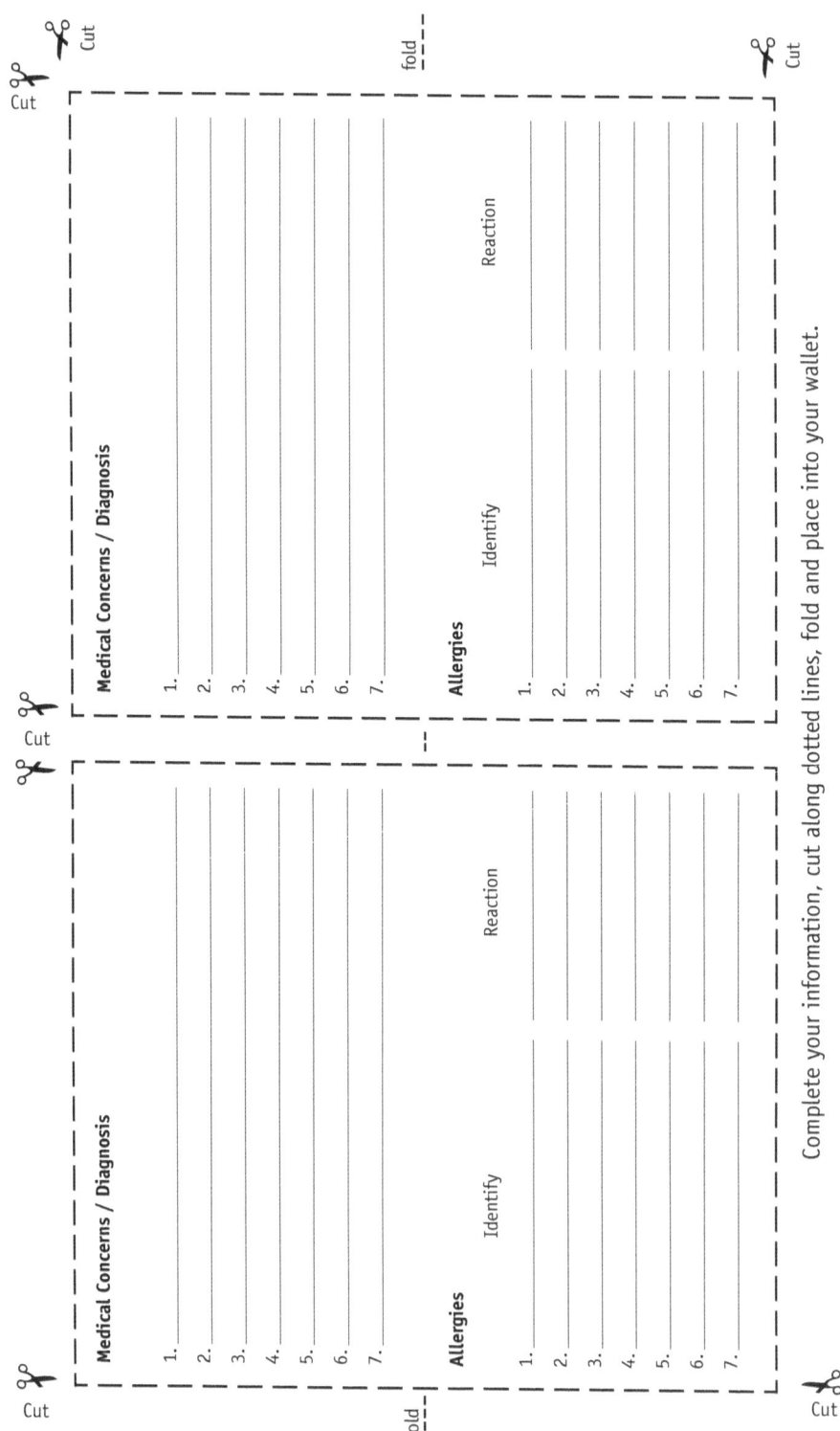

Medical Concerns / Diagnosis

1.
2.
3.
4.
5.
6.
7.

Allergies

Identify   Reaction

1.
2.
3.
4.
5.
6.
7.

Medical Concerns / Diagnosis

1.
2.
3.
4.
5.
6.
7.

Allergies

Identify   Reaction

1.
2.
3.
4.
5.
6.
7.

fold

Cut

Cut

Cut

Cut

Cut

Complete your information, cut along dotted lines, fold and place into your wallet.

ABOUT THE AUTHOR

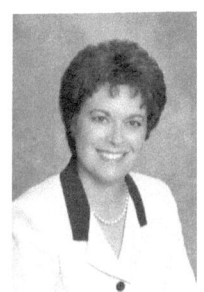

For over 33 years, Gloria A. Lopez has worked with children with disabilities, with their families and with adults who were diagnosed with medical conditions later in life. The Personal Medical Journal grew out of her experience and is designed to help you, or your caregiver, take control of your medical needs.

The first version of the Journal was created for her son, Michael, who was born with Spina Bifida, a neural tube birth defect. It continues to help her keep track of Michael's extensive medical information, eliminating the need for memorizing and reiterating his medical history. Additionally, it provides medical professionals easy and accurate access to important information in an emergency. She also used the journal for her two daughters who, although healthy, now have a concise, easily accessible medical history.

Gloria has helped start several support groups, including a group for parents experiencing the trauma of having a newborn in a neonatal hospital unit and local community parent support groups. She has assisted in developing a program to mainstream children with disabilities into local school districts in Santa Clara County, California.

As a speaker, a medical conference planner, an advocate for child and parental rights, and a program developer on a community, state and national level, Gloria has been active with many issues affecting the disabled. She was a founder and Administrative Director of the Spina Bifida Association of California and continues to work with hospitals on disability awareness and program development.

Gloria has shown many families and individuals how to put together their own Personal Medical Journal to assist them in maintaining accurate records and to help them take a more active role in their medical care.

GLORIA ANN LOPEZ

www.ingramcontent.com/pod-product-compliance
Lightning Source LLC
Chambersburg PA
CBHW031834170526
45157CB00001B/293